Before the Store
A guide to knowing what's in your grocery cart

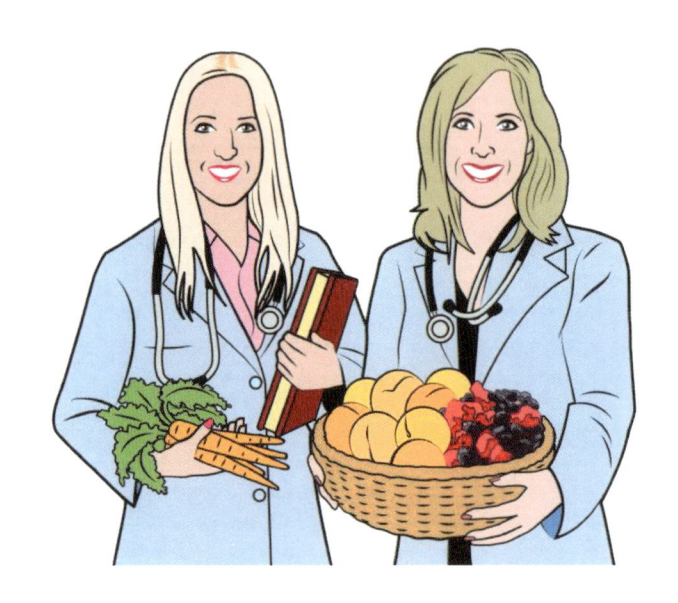

Jennifer Lucas, RN, MSN, FNP-BC

and

Jaclyn Taverna, RN, MSN, FNP-BC

Copyright © 2013 Jennifer Lucas and Jaclyn Taverna
All rights reserved.
ISBN-13: 978-1484094204
ISBN-10: 1484094204

Acknowledgements

To my dear husband, William Lucas, for spending years guiding me through this process and assisting me with photography, formatting, and editing. A special thanks to my family; Tom, Debbie, Mark, and Lauren Gambon for listening to my stories and food ideas over the years. Thank you to Dr. Andresen for sharing your knowledge. Thank you to Jackie for joining me on this project. May we educate, educate, educate. Thank you to all my patients, friends, and students for the motivation and stories that were needed during the last five years to write this guide.   *~ Jennifer*

Thank you to Jennifer Lucas who started this journey several years ago and pulled me onto her tractor for this educational, bumpy, and sometimes dusty ride through the farm. We made it! To my amazing family, especially my mom, Jane Lynch, thank you for your unconditional love and support. A heartfelt thank you to my sister, Joni Konstantelos, whose creative mind, humor, and writing style helped us maintain layman's language and kept us laughing throughout the whole writing process. And lastly, to all my patients, family, and friends who have helped challenge me to evaluate their ailments and discover how changes to their food sources could help them feel better.   *~ Jaclyn*

Jennifer and Jaclyn would like to acknowledge Deborah Ernst for spending countless hours editing this manuscript. This book would not have been possible without her dedication. Thank you to the professional organizations for their research and support. This book would not have been possible without Organic Consumers Association, Environmental Working Group, Marine Stewardship Council, Weston A. Price Foundation, Monterey Bay Aquarium, Cornucopia Institute, Non-GMO Project, Phil Howard from Michigan State, Sarah Ramsden, Glen Evans, Gina Lettiere, Farmer Alex, and the Loyola Student Farm.

~Jennifer and Jaclyn

Dedication

This book is dedicated to my dear grandpa Edward. I will always remember your farm stories and photos, as well as your always perceptive questions regarding changes in the food system.

~Jennifer

This book is dedicated to my children, Nathan and Julia. You are my most savory joys and my sweetest blessings. Thank you for your patience while mommy scans the aisles and picks apart ingredient lists.

~ Jaclyn

Contents

1	Fruits, Vegetables, and Herbs	14
2	Meat – Beef	18
3	Poultry – Chicken	21
4	Fish	25
5	Soy	29
6	Dairy	33
7	Eggs	43
8	In the Aisles	48
9	Beverages	72

Letters from the Nurses

Dear Fellow Shopper,

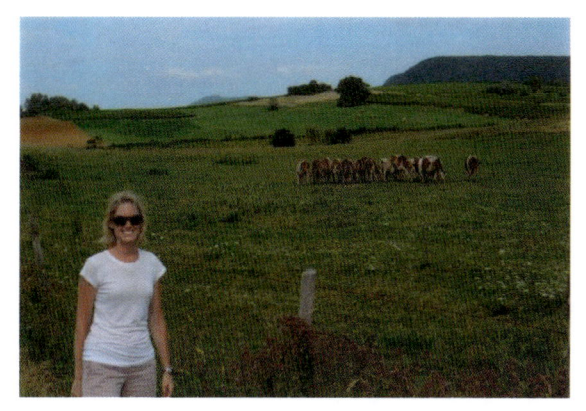

I truly believe that people are destined to do certain things in their lives. In my case it was written in the stars that I would, one day, educate about food and nutrition. My dad loves to tell a story from my childhood involving sweetened and unsweetened cereal. He came from a family of nine children who favored the sugary cereals on the market, and consequently, spent a great deal of time at the dentist having cavities filled. As adults, my parents decided that cereals with less sugar would be served to their children. One day, when I was about three years old, I witnessed a discussion between my parents after a box of sugary cereal surfaced in the house. I listened intently to their conversation and took my stand. I placed the new box of cereal into the trash. That moment was the beginning of my mission!

    I loved going grocery shopping with my mom as a young girl. She was selective about the ingredients she purchased. Meanwhile, the brightly colored packaging burst with promises of purity, health, and happiness. Mom cautioned me about buying something based on its glamorous appearance. Years later, I continue to apply my mom's lesson as I reach for raw honey and pure butter.

    Packaged foods we eat today are often a cluster of chemicals, preservatives, and fillers. These are methods manufacturers use to enhance the flavor, color, consistency, and taste of the product to make it resemble a "pure food" from nature. However, these methods have been linked to an increase in healthcare consumption and chronic diseases.

My journey continued as a graduate nursing student at Loyola University Chicago. I was experiencing frequent headaches, stomachaches, weight gain, and an overall lack of energy. I blamed it on stress, but that didn't seem right. After visits with an integrative medicine physician and through research, I found information on genetically modified organisms (GMO's), pesticides, and antibiotics. My head was spinning. Since "we are what we eat," I started investigating what exactly *I am* eating.

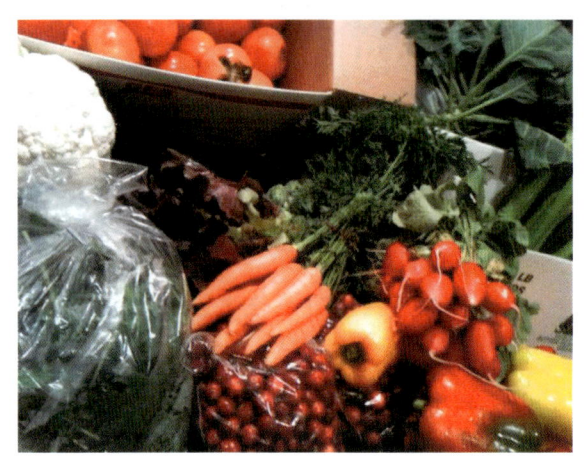

This guide pulls back the curtain to reveal what's in your food. This guide provides a brief history of foods, explains industry terminology, and helps you make better decisions as a consumer. Through education and informed decision-making at the grocery store, we can improve our health and our quality of life, one bite at a time.

~Jennifer

Dear Fellow Shopper,

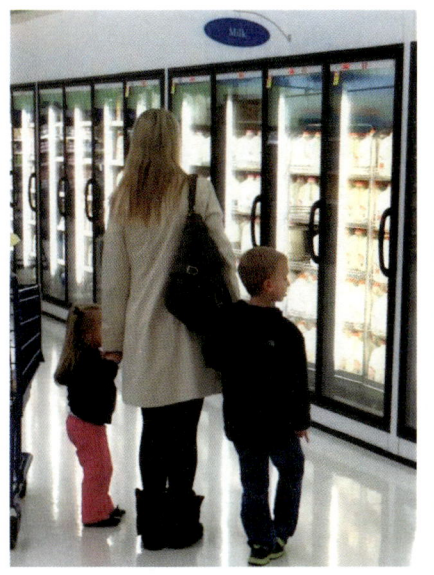

As a mother of two young children, I am oftentimes overwhelmed by my maternal duty to do what is right for my children, to protect them from harm, and to give them the best possible start in their lives. Standing in the refrigerated section of the grocery store, I feel the same sense of overwhelming responsibility, torn between choosing the "healthiest" options for my children and my pocketbook. As my eyes drift from one brand of milk to the next, organic vs. non-organic, the prices range from $1.79/gallon to $7.00/gallon. I can't help but think of my young children; innocent, healthy, pure, undeveloped. They are a blank canvas for a beautiful painting, an empty baby book waiting for milestones and memories. Will the milk I choose really make that much of a difference?

Organic had once been the standard for human nutrition. However, today's conventional farming, which includes the use of harmful pesticides, has contributed to the rise in the resistance to antibiotics, food allergies, and asthma.[1] Cancer rates have risen by a whopping 50% since 1950[2], cardiovascular disease is now the number one killer of women[3], and, in the United States, by 2020, more than half of all adults will have or be at risk for Type 2 diabetes.[4] It can be argued that technology as well as diagnostic tests and procedures have aided in the more thorough identification of such disease states, but it is undeniable that extreme changes in our food system have also played a major role. Young girls are developing at a much more rapid pace than ten years ago, menstruating as early as age 8![5] Their breasts are developing earlier, and are larger than ever before. Young boys are reaching puberty two years earlier than in the past.[6] One in 50 children has some type of autism, and other emotional/behavioral conditions, such as ADHD, are on the rise.[7]

For me, grocery shopping was once an enjoyable endeavor…that is, until I became a nutritionist, a nurse practitioner, and a mother. A treasure hunt for dinner recipe ingredients and snack foods has turned into a struggling swim through a murky swamp where I feel blinded, tricked, and robbed. As I maneuver the aisles, I am plagued by questions: Why are people so sick? Why are people so overweight? Which fruits do I need to buy organic? Why is high-fructose corn syrup so bad? Should I care about bovine growth hormones? Why can't I buy everything I need in one store?

So here I stand in the dairy department, my mind juggling between my credit card bills, my monthly expenses, and my children's health and well-being. The banker on my left shoulder tells me to purchase the sale-priced milk. After all, my kids are still eating processed macaroni and cheese, chicken nuggets, and chips. The nutritionist and nurse practitioner on my right, however, scream loudly about growth hormones; genetically modified organisms; as well as the filthy, in-humane conditions of factory farms.

If you are like me, and often find yourself with this dilemma, this book is for you! This grocery guide is aimed at helping you choose the healthiest options and move on with your day feeling a little less guilty. Don't Stress!! The more you consult this guide during grocery trips and meal planning, you will quickly pick up on marketing scams and questionable ingredients, but, most importantly, you will trust which brands are the best for your family. Not only will your family be healthier, you will feel better knowing you are helping them to become the best they can be, from the inside out. Change is not easy, but like anything in life; it happens one step at a time.

~Jaclyn

4

Letters from our Readers

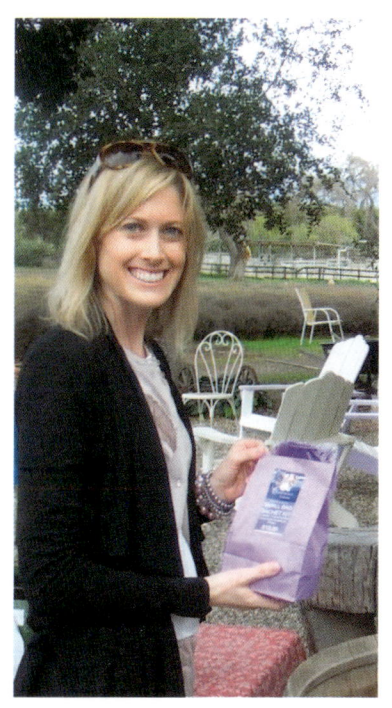

We would love to hear from you. If you would like to share information about a family farm, your favorite brand, or have questions about certain foods, email us at **healthyfarmplateyou@gmail.com.**

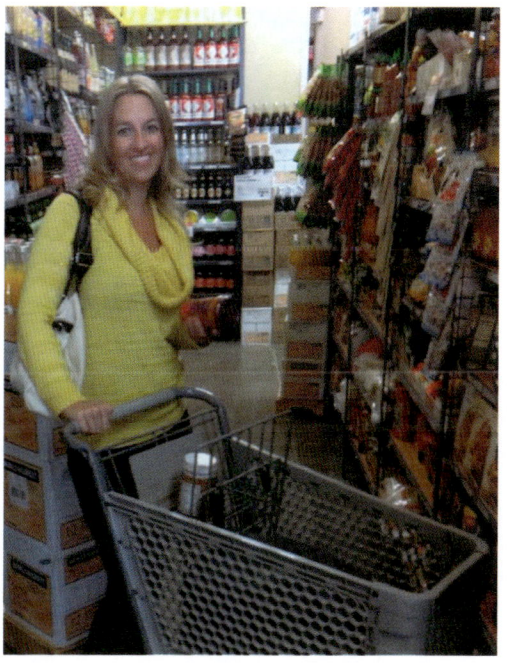

Introduction

The health and wellness industry has become a profitable business. Analysts predict the global industry, in 2017, will top $1 trillion.[8] With 35% of adults[9] and 17% of children and adolescents[10] of the U.S. population considered overweight or obese, promises of a quick slim-down and ways to get healthier are everywhere. While it is true that a well-balanced diet, low in saturated fat, contributes to the overall quality of our health, what if the chicken and veggies I am serving for dinner are actually contributing to weight gain, cancer, emotional disorders, and antibiotic resistance?

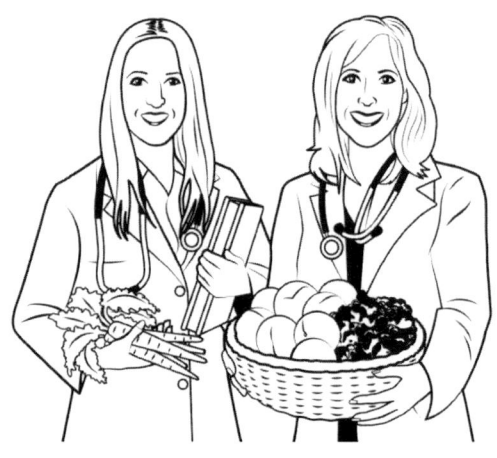

    The way in which food is grown and produced in the United States has changed dramatically since World War II. Many traditional farmers are turning off their plows and hanging up their overalls in search of careers outside the home. In addition, our households have changed; both parents work outside the home and our children are busier than ever, leaving little time to eat dinner, let alone make dinner. We have become a grab-and-go society; but, what exactly are we grabbing?

    Technology has brought many advances to our society today, as a result, greatly transforming the food industry. Concentrated Animal Feeding Operations (CAFO's) have replaced traditional farms, mass producing meat, produce and dairy. Chemicals, preservatives, and fillers have been added to our food to enhance the appearance and taste, as well as to make it last longer. Have you ever stopped and asked yourself, or someone else, what exactly a preservative is? What exactly are these chemicals being added to our foods? Furthermore, what are these additives doing to our bodies?

If we want to eat "healthy," shouldn't we understand what we are eating? Cows have survived for hundreds of years eating grass. Would you be shocked if I told you that, today, some cows eat corn, antibiotics, and gummy bears?[11] Yes, gummy bears! Cows are given hormone injections to make them produce more milk.[12] Chickens are given antibiotics to stave off infection from deplorable living conditions.[13] Our plant life is being genetically altered to include a pesticide gene into the seed of the plant.[14] If the old adage "We are what we eat" is true, then, what in the heck are we truly eating?

To answer this question, we have to go to the source. We need to do a background check on the food we consume. Where did that chicken come from? Did it eat grass or corn? Was the corn genetically modified? Where did the cow graze? What were the conditions? Was it injected with growth hormones, fed antibiotics, or sprayed with pesticides? And what about fish? Did that fish swim in a stream of industrial waste products, cleaning product residue, or plastics? Appetizing, isn't it?! Green leafy vegetables have many vital nutrients, but what if they are sprayed with pesticides, insecticides, or herbicides? What if they are genetically engineered?

Okay, by now, you are dizzy, a little sick to your stomach, and ready to reach for the potato chips, candy bar, or take-out menu. Don't! Put the take-out menu away and don't stop reading! We created this grocery guide to provide you with the knowledge necessary to make informed decisions about what to put in your cart and what to feed your family. As we began researching food and their sources, we discovered that there are many "ingredients" in processed foods, fruits, vegetables, dairy, meats, and fish that are actually contributing to illnesses. We were shocked to learn the number of additives that are in so many of our foods and disheartened by the negative effects they can have on our bodies. The light bulb went on as we did more research…no wonder our society is overweight, tired, emotionally drained, and that the incidence of disease is climbing faster than a Boeing 737 upon takeoff.

Our investigation all came back to one main conclusion: it is all about food *sources*. If the meat we eat comes from a traditional farm, where antibiotics and growth hormones are not used, where the food grown is pure and natural, we can worry less and enjoy that steak more! Similarly, if our produce was grown in a garden with clean soil, without being drenched in pesticides, or other harmful chemicals, we can enjoy our salads worry free. In other words, if we have to eat our vegetables, we might as well ensure they are the healthiest they can be.

So...What *should* I eat??? The answer to that question lies in the pages ahead. In this book, you will find an easy to use guide with fun icons that tell you what foods to look for, which ones to limit, and the most preferable brands to purchase. Our recommendations are based on the work of many nonprofit organizations and cover the hot topics of today.

The food industry is dynamic and information regarding food is constantly changing and evolving. For the most up-to-date information, please visit our website: **www.healthyfarmplateyou.com.**

A Word about Community Supported Agriculture (CSA)

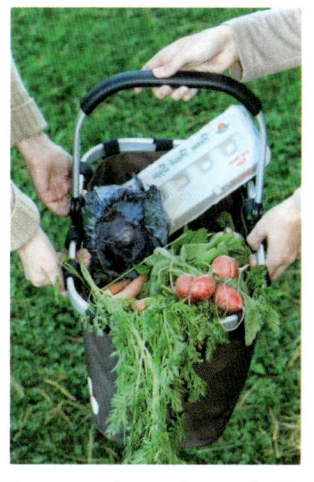

We love the on-site pick-up options at department stores. We can do all of our shopping on-line and have it ready at the store to pick up when we get there. Why can't we do this with our groceries? As it turns out, WE CAN! The website www.localharvest.org allows us to purchase food just like our department store experience, only from a CSA. CSA, short for Community Supported Agriculture, is just a fancy name for buying direct from the farm. Once on the local harvest website, click on the CSA tab, type in your zip code, and, like magic, all the farms that deliver fresh produce, meat, dairy, and eggs to your areas are listed. Even living in a major United States city or suburb, we were able to have farm-fresh food delivered to our area. The first Wednesday of every month, we stop by the "host house" in our area, usually a house or business, and pick up our groceries! In the bag, are different cuts of meat, individually wrapped, and labeled. Once you eat meat from a CSA, you will taste the difference. Our families and friends think we are the best cooks and while we agree, we also know the secret is out, grass-fed meat tastes better! This starts the conversation that not only finding the right source for meat helps it taste better, it's healthier too. Purchasing meat from a family farm through a CSA is easier than ever before.

Note: When finding a CSA, ask the farmers about their farming practices (explained later in the book) to ensure you are buying the healthiest products.

Farmers Market

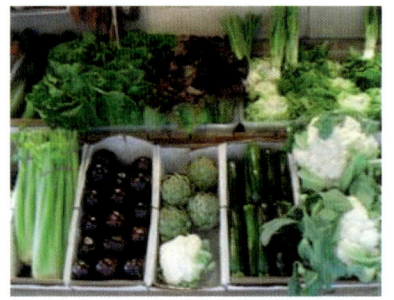

For us, a Saturday morning in the spring, summer, and fall would not be complete without spending time at the farmers market! We just feel healthier buying our produce and eggs from the people who actually grow or raise it. It is important, however, to get to know your farmer before you make a commitment. Know what questions to ask before you "put a ring on him!" For example: How do you grow or care for your tomatoes, corn, beans, lettuce, chickens, etc.? Ask the farmer to explain his or her method of farming instead of asking "yes" or "no" questions. Ask your farmer about where the produce was grown and when it was picked. Produce should be picked that day or the day before, and should not have travelled across the country. That is the whole point of a farmers market; buy local so it's fresh. Ask your farmer about suggestions for storing, preserving, and preparing a particular food. Also, don't be afraid of veggies you have never tried before. As a kid, I hated Brussels sprouts; after learning different ways to cook them, however, they have become one of my favorite vegetables.

Farmers, like other small business owners, like to talk about their work. They will gladly explain how they care for and feed their animals, tell you if they use pesticides during the growing season, and identify each season's challenges and opportunities, such as weather, soil, and insects. It is important to note that not all *organic* farmers have the USDA organic sticker. Like most anything involving the government, there is a lot of thick, bureaucratic red tape to go through to get that pretty little sticker. But, in this case, it is a good thing, so don't be afraid to ask!

Change

Implementing change in the way we grocery shop can be a difficult process. Change elicits different emotions: mistrust, apprehension, and anxiety. It is natural to become defensive in justifying the products we purchase and lovingly feed to our families. Keep in mind the following points as you try to slowly adjust the way you grocery shop to incorporate healthier choices for your family.

1. Pattern. Most people have their own grocery shopping pattern. They go to their favorite stores and are familiar with the stores' layouts and the products they carry. As you gain more knowledge about food, CSA's, farmers markets, and organic web-stores, you will be able to change or add these healthier options into your pattern of grocery shopping. We get our meat every month from the CSA, produce from the farmers market, and I know which stores carry my favorite type of organic milk and have the best price. We still shop *"the aisles"* of our favorite stores for our staples and pantry items.

2. Price. What do you mean I have to pay more? In the end, our advice is to buy the healthiest food that you can afford, for yourself and your family. We have to remind ourselves that food costs money and *real* food costs more. However, in the end, *real* food costs less than medications, hospital bills, and doctor visits. Our philosophy is that you either pay for pure, healthy food now, or pay for it later in the form of bills associated with chronic illnesses or time spent away from work, loved ones, and hobbies. So, we've decided to shop at the farmers market, join a CSA, and make more of our own meals.

3. Time. At first, it takes more time but, then it gets easier (see the pattern section above). Our advice is to implement one change per month. Working full time and raising a family, we slowly and steadily implemented the changes.

This is the plan we used for our first year of change.

January:	Research CSA's.
February:	Sign-up for a CSA.
March:	Make more meals at home with the CSA meat.
April:	Plant herbs.
May:	Research farmers markets in the area.
June:	Go to the farmers market every other week.
July:	Buy a bread machine and make homemade bread.
August:	Make homemade broth.
September:	Freeze local in-season fruit for the winter.
October:	Make fresh-squeezed orange juice.
November:	Research organic milk by price and store.
December:	Purchase pantry staples from web-store, such as *Green Polka-Dot-Box*.

It is three years later, and we have made over 30 changes!!! We have lost weight and have more energy and time! It only takes one change a month!

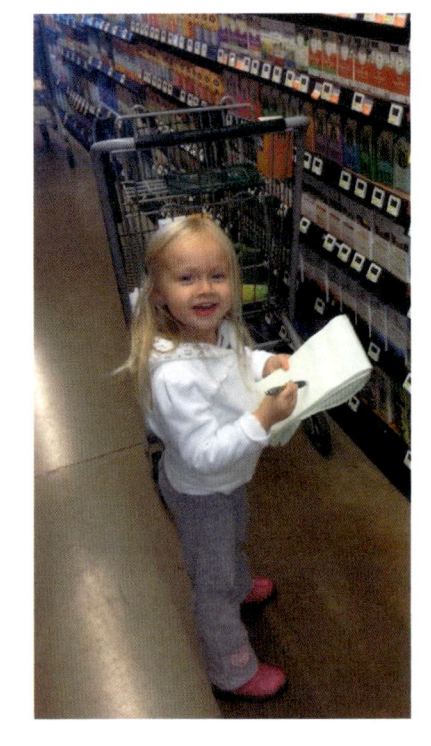

Disclaimer

The information presented in this book is offered for educational and informational purposes only and is not to be constructed as personal medical advice. You should consult with your health care provider regarding medical care for yourself or others.

We are not endorsing any brands, nor are we affiliated with any of the companies noted in this book. We do not advocate cutting all the foods in the "Limit" categories from your lives, but, instead, to practice moderation. We do not believe that we can eat by an "all-or-nothing" principle.

KEY

Look for the friendly nurses throughout the pages to find recommendations.

Food history - what changes occurred in our food throughout the years and what is currently happening.

Health implications.

Limit these foods in your cart and in your home!

The quick-tip guy! When in doubt, follow his advice.

Money saving tips!

Color Code: Throughout the book you will find brands of food in **Green** and **Purple** font. According to the Weston A. Price Foundation, **Green** brands are **Best** options at the store and **Purple** brands are **Good** options.

1. Fruits & Vegetables

Buy Fresh   Buy Local   Buy Organic

For thousands of years, fruits and vegetables have grown out in the wild. People used to eat them by simply gathering nature's supply off the trees and plants. These early humans had to spend many of their waking hours searching for these gems, because Mother Nature's production was not always consistent. Many fruits were only available in the springtime, and vegetables, being the stem, root, or leaf of a plant, were harvested all year. Luckily, people learned to use the seeds Mother Nature provided and saved them from year to year. Methods, such as crop rotation, kept the soil rich and reduced pests; chemicals or pesticides were not used. Those who still use these methods are known as "organic farmers" and their produce is called "organic." Many farmers grow their crops organically, even though they are not labeled with a USDA certified organic label. The USDA organic labeling process is expensive, costing farmers anywhere from $5,000-$25,000 every five years, on average.[15]

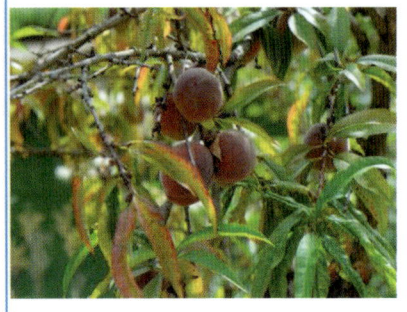

According to the U.S. Environmental Protection Agency (EPA), over 1 billion tons of pesticides are used in the U.S. every year.[16] Furthermore, there are 350,000 pesticide products registered.[17] Today, most produce grown in the United States is sprayed with pesticides. This produce is rarely labeled with terms like "conventional" or "non-organic." Scientists discovered that by designing a seed with pesticide resistant properties, when the crop is sprayed with chemicals, the weeds will die, but not the plant.[18] These crops are called genetically modified organisms (GMO's). These GMO seeds are on the Environmental Protection Agency's (EPA) pesticide list because they contain pesticides.[19]

Pesticides are designed to kill living things and accomplish this by causing nerve damage in the brains of bees and pests. These pesticides are toxic and many can cause cancer, birth defects, neural disorders, and other health problems.[20]

Many types of produce are imported from other countries so that we can eat them during the off-growing seasons. Produce is irradiated when it is exported and imported, meaning it has been given high doses of radiation to kill microbes in the food.[21] Unfortunately, the radiation also kills enzymes and damages nutrients. So, in short, buy local!

Questions to Ask

1. Was the produce sprayed with pesticides throughout the growing season or at any time?
2. Is this a GMO fruit or vegetable?
3. When was it picked?
4. How many miles did the produce travel from the farm to table?

What Should I Look For?
- Local produce from a family farm, through a CSA, farmers market, food co-op, or grocery store
- Produce that isn't sprayed with pesticides throughout the growing season
- A sticker code that starts with a number "**9**" (organic)
- In-season produce
- Follow the Environmental Working Group (EWG) chart (pg. 16), if you decide not to buy all organic. EWG's chart shows fruits and vegetables that should be purchased organic due to the high levels of pesticide residue on that particular fruit or vegetable.

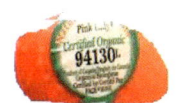

⚠️ What Should I Limit?

- 🍏 GMO produce—This produce has a sticker on its skin with a five-digit number that starts with an "**8**" (genetically engineered).
- 🍏 Produce is grown as non-organic and organic. Scientists in the lab, have genetically modified (GMO) Zucchini, yellow crookneck squash, sweet corn, and Hawaii papaya[22] to make them resistant to pesticides. Currently, scientists are developing more GMO produce.
- 🍏 Produce that is not in season; it is likely imported
- 🍏 Sticker on the skin with **four** numbers (sprayed with pesticides)
- 🍏 Produce from other countries, especially non-organic
- 🍏 Bruised produce

Buy from a local farm to get the ripest produce with the least amount of handling! In the store, look at the sticker: "Dine with **9, 4** no more, walk straight past **8**".

Grow your own! Buy in-season produce and can, freeze, or dehydrate (dry) extras for the year.

Environmental Working Group (EWG) developed a guide. For the app, full report, and chart, go to www.ewg.org/foodnews.[23]

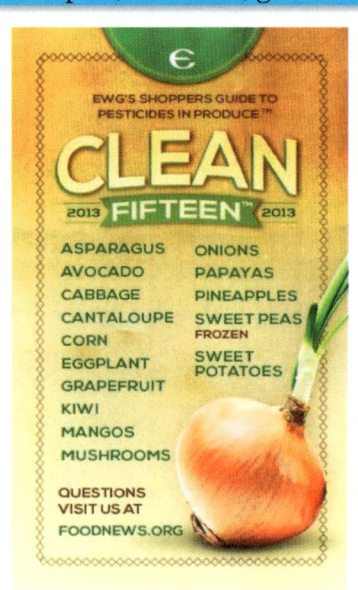

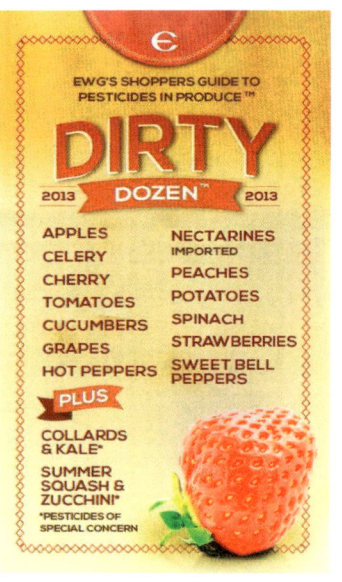

EWG'S SHOPPERS GUIDE TO PESTICIDES IN PRODUCE™

CLEAN FIFTEEN™ 2013
- ASPARAGUS
- AVOCADO
- CABBAGE
- CANTALOUPE
- CORN
- EGGPLANT
- GRAPEFRUIT
- KIWI
- MANGOS
- MUSHROOMS
- ONIONS
- PAPAYAS
- PINEAPPLES
- SWEET PEAS FROZEN
- SWEET POTATOES

QUESTIONS VISIT US AT FOODNEWS.ORG

EWG'S SHOPPERS GUIDE TO PESTICIDES IN PRODUCE™

DIRTY DOZEN™ 2013
- APPLES
- CELERY
- CHERRY TOMATOES
- CUCUMBERS
- GRAPES
- HOT PEPPERS
- NECTARINES IMPORTED
- PEACHES
- POTATOES
- SPINACH
- STRAWBERRIES
- SWEET BELL PEPPERS

PLUS
- COLLARDS & KALE*
- SUMMER SQUASH & ZUCCHINI*

*PESTICIDES OF SPECIAL CONCERN

Copyright © Environmental Working Group, www.ewg.org. Reprinted with permission.

Fruits & Vegetables (canned, dried, frozen)

What Should I Look For?

- Canned produce in water, in its own juice, or in light syrup.
- Cans labeled "BPA free."
- Organic frozen and dried fruits and vegetables

What Should I Limit?

- Corn syrup, sugar, or additives
- Cans containing BPA (not labeled that it contains BPA)

Example Brands to Buy for Canned

Bionaturae tomato products
Eden
Farmer's Market
Field Day
Lucini Tomatoes
Mediterranean Organic
Native Forest
Whole Foods (365)
Woodstock Farm

The Weston A. Price Foundation recommends the following brands. For more brands and suggestions, go to www.westonaprice.org.[24]

Example Brands to Buy

Aimee's Livin' Magic dried fruit
Bionaturae tomato products in glass jars
Blue Mountain Organics sea vegetables
Cascadian Farms frozen fruits and vegetables
Divine Organics sun-dried tomatoes
Eden crushed tomatoes in glass jars
Eden sea vegetables
Essential Living Foods dried fruit
Lucini tomatoes in glass jars
Mediterranean Organic sun-dried tomatoes
Miller's Organic Farm frozen peas

2. Meat (beef)

Local   Family Farm   Local

Traditional farming is known today as organic farming. On these farms; cows, chickens, pigs, and other animals are able to roam freely among valleys and pastures, eating naturally growing grass and vegetation. The discovery of GMO corn, antibiotics, and growth hormones has facilitated raising these animals indoors in order to speed up growth, maximizing the quantity of meat available to sell to markets and consumers.[25] Raising animals for food has become a profitable business for large corporations. These corporations purchase family farms and turn them into Concentrated Animal Feeding Operations (CAFO). In a CAFO, thousands of animals are in a metal building or outdoor pen with no room to move. The goal is for these animals to grow as quickly as possible so that they can be sent to market. The animals are injected and fed a variety of things to meet this goal. To produce more milk, some of the cows are injected with growth hormones (rBGH).[26] To gain weight, they are fed GMO corn and soybeans, fats, and antibiotics.[27] Cows are, by nature, meant to eat grass, so they become very sick with this unnatural diet.

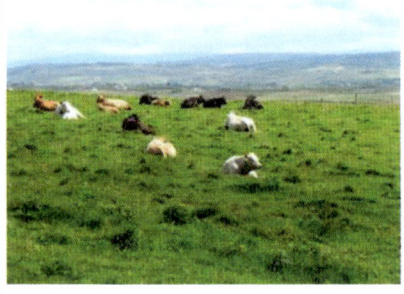

It is important to know what the animals are eating and how they are treated, as this directly impacts our health. When we consume animal products, we are actually eating what the animal ate. Remember, **We Are What We Eat**. On a molecular level, many things affect our cells. For example, growth hormones (rBGH) are linked to early development in females; less sperm in males; and cancers of the breast, prostate, and colon.[28] On the other hand, grass-fed cattle have meat lower in total fat and higher in omega fatty acids, which decreases inflammation.[29]

A Note on Organic Meat

There are such things as organic factory farms, where the animals still live on large farms without grazing on grass. The only difference is instead of eating GMO grains, they are eating organic grains. The health benefits do not dramatically improve if the meat is organic compared to non-organic.[30] Pasture time or time spent grazing in the pasture directly affects the nutritional profile of the meat. The best source for meat is directly from a family farm.

Questions to Ask

1. Did the cow eat grass or corn?
2. Was the cow given antibiotics for weight gain or for illness?
3. Does the meat contain additives, nitrites, or natural flavors?
4. If organic, did the meat come from a CAFO or a family farm?

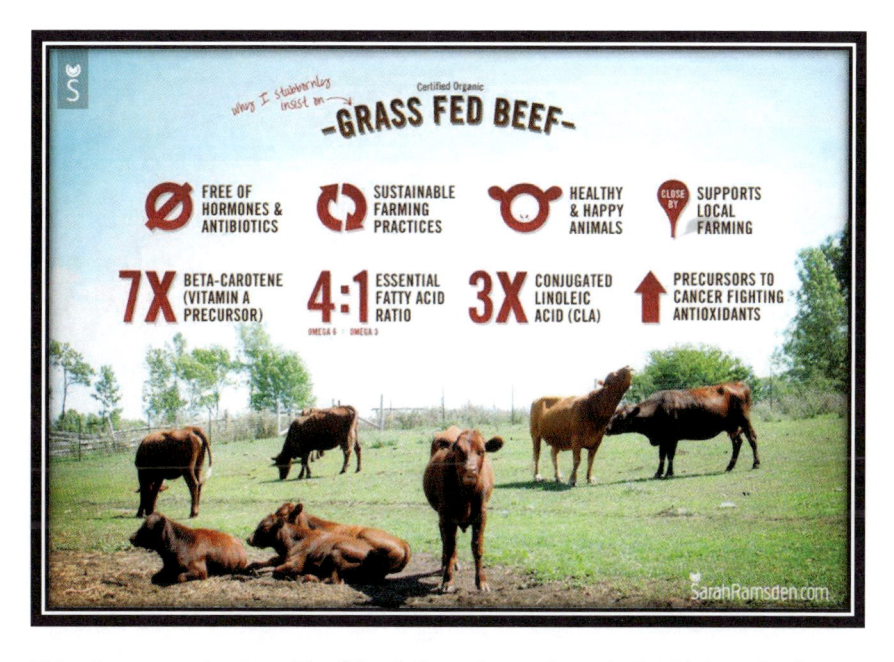

This picture was developed by ©Sarah Ramsden to show the health benefits from eating grass-fed beef. Sarah Ramsden, MA, CNP is a Holistic Nutritionist who helps people in Canada reinvent their health. Visit her website at http://www.sarahramsden.com/grass-fed-beef.[31]

What Should I Look for?

- Meat from a family farm through a CSA, farmers market, food Co-op, or local butcher.
- 100% grass-fed meat
- Grass-fed meat
- Organic meat

What Should I Limit?

- Growth hormones (rBGH), antibiotics, and corn-fed
- Additives, nitrites, natural flavors, hydrolyzed protein, and MSG

Terms such as "natural" are not regulated by the government. So, they do not have much meaning.[32]

Buy from a CSA or farmers market to save money and time!

To find brands in your area, go to **www.eatwild.com**. This website provides a list of grocery stores which sell "grass-fed" meats. For example, here is an abbreviated list for Chicago, IL.

| Crafthouse Market Goods | Dill Pickle Co-Op | Fox & Obel Market |
| South Pork Ranch | Mint Creek Farm | Tallgrass Beef |

The Weston A. Price Foundation recommends the following brands. For more brands and suggestions, go to www.westonaprice.org.[33]

Example Brands to Buy for Beef

Copper Creek Farms	Nature's Prime Organic Foods
Deck Family Farm	Niman Ranch
Good Earth Farms	Organic Grass-fed Beef Coalition
Miller's Biodiversity Farm	
Miller's Organic Farm	Organic Prairie
Mint Creek Farm	Trader Joe's

3. Poultry (chicken)

Local   Family Farm   Local

On the family farm, my great-grandmother's job was to care for the chickens. She let her chickens roam the open air, eat insects and table scraps, and reproduce naturally. At night, she made sure each and every one of them was in the chicken coop. She was especially proud of her chicken named "Lucy," as she lived to be twenty-one years old, while the average life expectancy of a chicken is fifteen to twenty years.

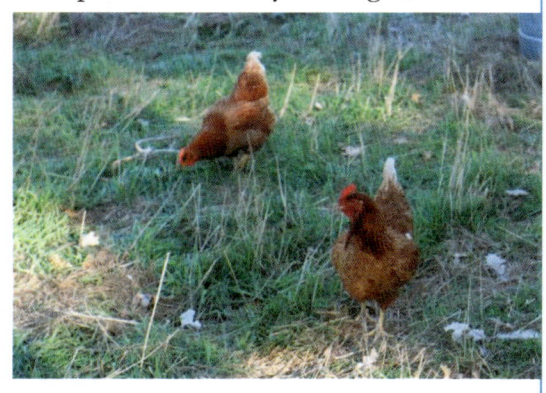

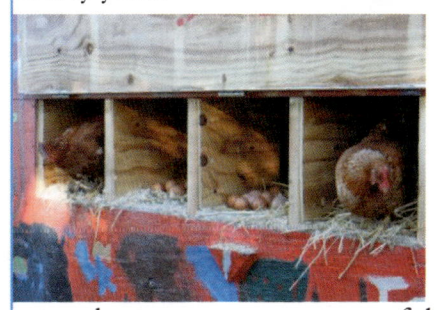

My great-grandmother would be shocked to know what I am about to share with you. In today's modern world, we consume a great deal of chicken. Unfortunately, in order to produce the large amount of chicken needed, these animals are no longer seen as creatures of the earth, but as a commodity without any rights. Chickens are exempt from the Humane Methods of Slaughter Act[34], so no laws protect them from harm. In the United States, about 7 billion chickens per year are sent to the slaughterhouse and 452 million hens are used for their eggs.[35] In Concentrated Animal Feeding Organizations (CAFO's), there are two kinds of chickens: broilers and laying hens.[36] In a CAFO, chickens that are used for meat (broilers) have been engineered to grow more than twice as large in less than half the time.[37] Their muscles and fat tissues grow faster than their bones, causing diseased and deformed birds. Chickens are now selectively bred to produce more breast meat at a lower cost. In fact, there is a genetically engineered chicken that is made to grow without feathers.[38] These types of birds are created to develop more quickly in order to move to the market faster. CAFO chickens live in a "modern-day" chicken coop: a metal building crammed with thousands of chickens. They are housed in tight spaces and fed antibiotics, corn, soy, and scraps to help them gain weight quickly.[39] These scraps are not the dinner left-overs my great-grandmother fed her chickens, but the scraps that are leftover from the CAFO's (processed feathers, feces, plastic pellets, meat and bone meal).[40] Thankfully, the government protects them from being injected with growth hormones.[41]

When chickens are seven weeks old, they are moved to the slaughterhouse.[42] Keep in mind that the average chicken lives to be fifteen years old. They are bathed in chlorine to kill the bacteria they collected while living in the CAFO.[43] This, however, is not always effective; the consumer, therefore, is subject to food poisoning. Before the chickens are put on the market, they are injected with a syringe full of a salty solution to plump them and make them taste like a chicken. We, in turn, ingest this salt solution, because there are binding agents in the solution which prevent the added salt and water from leaving the chicken.[44]

One of the major concerns is antibiotic resistance. Healthy and sick chickens are given antibiotics for weight gain and to keep them alive.[45] When we consume chicken, we are also being exposed to trace amounts of antibiotics. Furthermore, we are being exposed to the medications and foods that were given to the chicken for weight gain and, therefore, we, as consumers, may gain weight from these weight inducers.[46] On the other hand, when we consume organic, pasture-raised chickens that spent time in the pasture and ate an organic diet, we are consuming more omega-3s, and antioxidants, but less fat.[47]

Important Terms to Know

- Heritage: Domestic breeds that have been raised in a natural wild environment
- "Enhanced with up to 15% chicken broth": Infused with salt solution
- Antibiotic-Free/No Antibiotics: Did not receive antibiotics
- Pastured or Pasture-Raised: Chickens raised on grass instead of in closed barn
- Organic: No GMO feed mix, antibiotics or animal by-products; received some outdoor access. There is, however, no requirement for amount of time outside or location, therefore, some places have their "outdoor time" in a screened porch.
- No hormones given: hormones are not allowed in chickens, so this product is not better than another, it's only a marketing term.

Questions to Ask

1. Is the chicken from a CAFO or family farm?
2. Was the chicken able to be outdoors for exercise?
3. Does the poultry contain "natural flavors?"
4. What did the chicken eat?
5. Did the chicken live in a cage in a metal building or was it in a chicken coop, spending most of its time outside?
6. Was the chicken fed antibiotics for weight gain or for illness?

What Should I Look For?

Chicken from a family farm, through a CSA, farmers market, food co-op, local butcher, or grocery store
These terms: Pastured, pasture raised or organic and pastured.

What Should I Limit?

Non-organic

These terms: natural, free-range, and cage-free (not regulated)

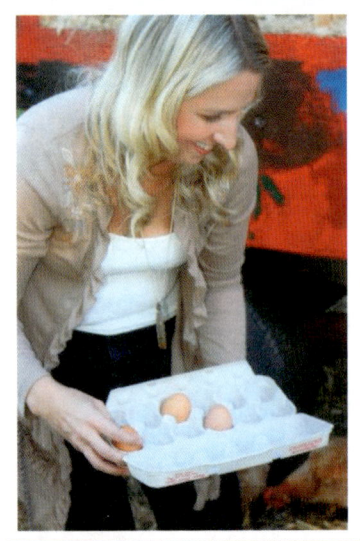

Buy from a CSA, farmers market, or directly from the famer.

Buy from a CSA to save money and time

The Weston A. Price Foundation recommends the following brands. For more brands and suggestions, go to www.westonaprice.org.[48]

Example Brands to Buy

Bell & Evans	Smart Organic	Trader Joe's
Niman Ranch	Smart Chicken	Prairie Pride

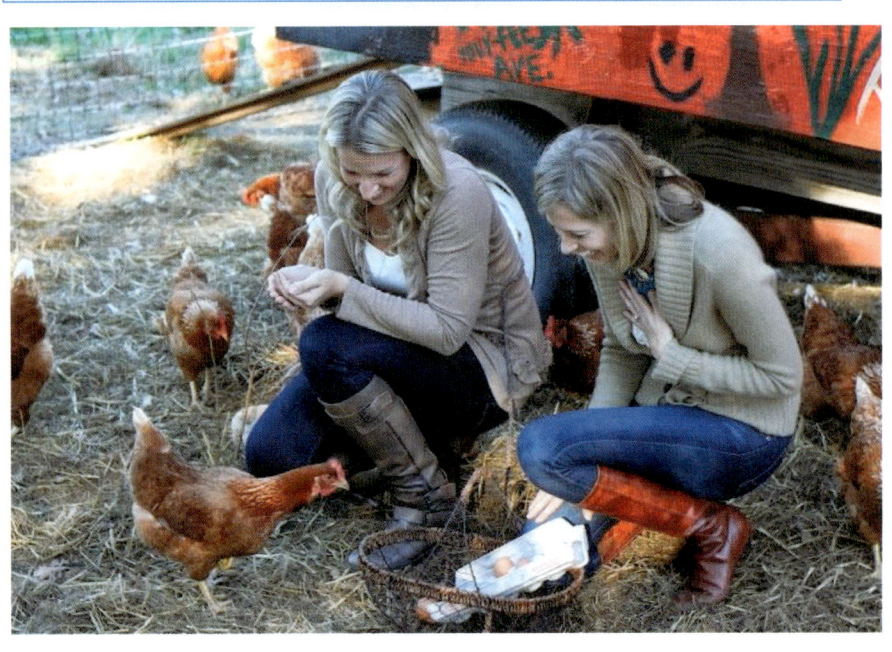

Grazing chickens in the pasture equals happy chickens

24

3. Fish

Know Your Fish

Historically, fishermen went fishing with their nets or fishing poles. Today, most fishermen are emptying the oceans by using GPS monitors, longlines with billions of hooks, and thirty-mile-long nets.[49] Longline fishing kills fish, along with millions of other sea creatures. Fish living in the ocean are labeled *wild caught,* while fish living in fish farms are labeled *farmed raised.* Some farm-raised fish is better due to the pollutants found in wild fish, while others are unhealthy and better to buy wild. Most fish farms are treated with herbicides to prevent water plant growth, fed pellets to dye the fish, fed GMO grains and contain parasitic sea lice.[50]

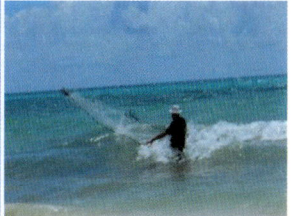

A company designed a GMO salmon, which grows faster than normal salmon, by making it constantly produce growth hormones.[51] When we consume this fish, then we are, in turn, ingesting these hormones. Sadly, GMO salmon does not have to be labeled as such.

For many years, pollutants have filled the oceans and lakes as a result of companies dumping toxic wastes into the water, oil spills, littering, and raw sewage. Fish are filters, as they swim through the water and, therefore, pick up PCB's (Polychlorinated Biphenyls) and mercury.[52] As the big fish eat the smaller fish, the big fish acquire the toxins from the smaller fish. This is why it is advisable to eat smaller fish to avoid a larger accumulation of toxins.

Farmed fish are more likely to carry increased levels of toxic chemicals and heavy metals that are known to cause such conditions as birth defects, miscarriages, immune disorders, learning disabilities, and various types of cancer.[53] Farmed fish is higher in saturated fat, toxic chemicals, and antibiotics.[54] There are also health consequences from eating wild-caught fish with environmental pollutants. Fish high in mercury and pollution toxins can cause nerve damage, miscarriages, learning disabilities, birth deformities, and cancers in humans.[55]

Questions to Ask

1. Is the fish wild or farmed?
2. Does the fish contain high amounts of mercury and PCB's?
3. How was the fish caught?

What Should I Look For?

- Follow the Monterey Bay Aquarium Seafood Watch Guide (pg. 27-28). Purchase fish labeled **green** or **yellow**
- Fish labeled **"wild fish" or "wild caught"**
- Canned light tuna (less mercury)
- Look for the Marine Stewardship Council (MSC) ecolabel in supermarkets, drug/nutritional supplement stores, and restaurants.

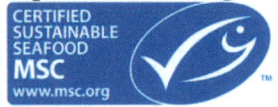

What Should I Limit?

- Servings of fish labeled **red**
- Farmed fish: shrimp, tuna, and salmon
- Large fish high in mercury and PCB's, such as tuna, shark, red snapper, king mackerel, swordfish, and tilefish
- Albacore ("white") tuna (higher in mercury)
- Organic seafood (likely farm-raised)

Follow the Monterey Bay Aquarium Seafood Watch guide. We have not found fish options labeled "GMO-free", therefore we recommend following the Seafood Watch guide.

The healthiest fish is going to cost more, so try to find it on sale.

Example Brands of Canned Tuna to Purchase

| Bar Harbor | Wild Planet | Sea Fare Pacific |

The Monterey Bay Aquarium's Seafood Watch® program helps consumers and businesses purchase seafood that is fished or farmed in ways that minimize their impact on the environment. By following their guidelines on the Seafood Watch website, app or pocket guide, grocers can commit to sourcing only sustainable seafood.[56]

*The pocket guide gets updated twice a year so download the app for up-to-date recommendations. Go to Seafoodwatch.org

Fall/Winter 2013 Central Seafood Watch Guide (Modified Version)[57]

Best Choices: well managed, caught or farmed in environmentally responsible ways

Arctic Char (farmed)
Bass: Striped (US hook & line, farmed)
Catfish (US)
Clams, Mussels, Oysters
Cod: Pacific (US)
Crab: Dungeness & Stone
Halibut: Pacific (US)
Lobster: Spiny (CA, FL & Mexico)
Perch: Yellow (Lake Erie)
Salmon (AK)
Sardines: Pacific (Canada & US)
Scallops (farmed)
Shrimp: Pink (OR)
Tilapia (Ecuador & US)
Trout: Rainbow (US farmed)
Tuna: Albacore/White canned (Canada & US troll, pole)
Tuna: Skipjack/Light canned (US troll, pole)
Tuna: Yellowfin (US troll, pole)
Whitefish: Lake (Lake Michigan trap net)
Whitefish: Lake (Lakes Superior & Huron)

Good Alternatives: some concerns with how they are caught or farmed

Basa/Pangasius/Swai	**Tilapia** (China & Taiwan)
Cod: Pacific (US trawl)	**Trout: Lake** (Lakes Huron & Superior)
Crab: Blue	
Crab: King (US)	**Tuna: Albacore/White canned** (US longline)
Flounders, Soles (US Pacific)	
Grouper: Red (US Gulf of Mexico)	**Tuna: Skipjack/Light canned** (imported troll, pole, and US longline)
Lobster: American	
Mahi Mahi (US)	**Tuna: Yellowfin** (imported troll, pole and US longline)
Salmon (CA, OR & WA wild)	
Scallops (wild)	**Whitefish: Lake** (Lake Erie)
Shrimp (Canada & US wild)	**Whitefish: Lake** (Lake Michigan gillnet)
Squid (US)	
Swordfish (US)	

Avoid: overfished or strong concerns with how they are caught or farmed

Abalone (China & Japan)	**Squid** (imported)
Caviar, Sturgeon (imported wild)	**Swordfish** (imported)
	Trout: Lake (Lake Michigan)
Cod: Pacific (imported)	**Tuna: Albacore/White canned** (except Canada & US troll, pole and US longline)
Crab: Red King (Russia)	
Lobster: Spiny (Brazil)	
Mahi Mahi (imported)	**Tuna: Bluefin**
Orange Roughy	**Tuna: Skipjack/Light canned** (except troll, pole, & US longline)
Salmon: Atlantic (farmed)	
Shark	
Shrimp (imported)	**Tuna: Yellowfin** (except troll, pole and US longline)
Snapper: Red (US)	

© 2013, Monterey Bay Aquarium Foundation

5. Soy

Organic

As a child, my family enjoyed blueberry picking every summer. The berries were so delicious that I always ate as many as I put into the bucket! We also loved picking strawberries in the spring and apples in the fall. There were soybean fields farther down the country road, and I wondered why we didn't pick these. My mom explained that the farmers planted soybeans to put nitrogen back into the soil so that the soil would be ready for corn to be planted the next year. The soybeans were meant to be plowed under the soil as green manure and not to be used for food.

In fact, soybeans cannot be consumed in the field, like blueberries, since they must be cooked or fermented before eating.[58] This, however, has been known for three millennia, when the Chinese realized the poisonous toxins in the bean could be neutralized with cooking or fermenting.[59] Once they discovered this, foods made from soybeans, such as, tofu, tempeh, soy sauce, miso, and natto, could be enjoyed.

There are many articles today that say we all consume too much soy. At first, I had a difficult time believing this, considering I do not usually drink soy lattes or consume soy burgers or tofu. So, one day, I walked into my pantry and started reading ingredient lists. I made a pile of all my foods that contain soy oil or soy lecithin. Boy, was I surprised! Even my organic products contained these ingredients. I started pulling the chicken and pork out of my refrigerator, and realized these animals were fed soy protein as well. Even my chocolate lab, Julius, was eating soy in his dog food! In the United States, soybean oil makes up 80% of all the oils on the market.[60] If the label says just 'vegetable oil,' there is a good chance that it is soy.[61] In other words, it is basically in everything. Most of us are eating small amounts of soy in almost every meal and snack we have throughout the day.

In our research, we discovered four main points to keep in mind:

1. Food *can* be labeled organic if it contains at least 95% of organic ingredients.[62] This means that up to 5% of ingredients can be non-organic. The soy ingredients, therefore, that are GMO and sprayed with pesticides can be added to organic foods.
2. Ninety-three percent of soybeans grown in the United States are GMO![63] Shocked? We are. This means that we are not only eating soy ingredients on a daily basis, we are eating GMO soy.
3. Soy lecithin (produced from soybean oil) is used to make food last longer on the grocery shelves as well as to hold ingredients together. Soy lecithin is found in ice cream, trail mix, crackers, cookies, cereal, candy, vitamins, alcohol, sports drinks, pizza toppings, seafood, diet products, margarine, salad dressing, infant formula, and much, much more.
4. Companies are constantly researching new soy products. It is a multi-billion-dollar business. For example, a company in Iowa has developed a variety of soybeans so that the texture of the soy protein is more "meat-like."[64]

There are many studies that cite both the health benefits as well as the health concerns of soy. Some studies say that soy protects the heart, while others say too much soy leads to health problems. Many health experts believe the average American consumes too much soy, especially modern-day soy ingredients (soy protein, soy lecithin, soy protein isolate, soy oil, etc.). This leads to an imbalance within the body, because soy is a precursor to estrogen. As a result, consuming large amounts of soy may lead to a decrease in libido; inhibit ovulation; and contribute to cancer, digestive problems, hormone disruption, and thyroid disease.[65] What about allergies? We need to ask ourselves, does exposure to these soy ingredients, in nearly every food product, lead to food allergies? Does GMO soy lead to food allergies? Time, and further research, will tell.

The bottom line is that soy should be consumed in moderation and it should be of the fermented variety. Fermented soy does not cause the health consequences mentioned above. Enjoy soy in moderation.

According to Dr. Weil, holistic health expert and founder of the Arizona Center for Integrative Medicine, this means 1-2 servings per day. One serving is equal to ½ cup tofu or tempeh, 1 cup soymilk, ½ cup cooked edamame, or 1 ounce of soy nuts.[66]

Fermented Soy	Non-fermented Soy
Miso	Unfermented Soy Products:
Natto	Soymilk
Tempeh	Tofu
Pickled Tofu	Textured soy protein
Soy Sauce (fermented traditionally)	Soy infant formula
Tamari	

Questions to Ask

1. Is it made with GMO soy and grown with pesticides?
2. Does it contain GMO soy ingredients such as soy protein, soy protein isolate, or textured vegetable protein?
3. Is it fermented or non-fermented soy?

What Should I Look For?

If you are going to consume soy products, follow the Cornucopia Institute's chart for the best choices. Buy brands rated "5" or "4," if not available, then "3" or "2."

Have more servings of fermented soy than non-fermented soy

What Should I Limit?

Soy ingredients: soy protein, soy protein isolate, etc.

Products rated "0", "1," or "Private Label" on the Cornucopia Institute's chart

Use the chart below as a guide.

Buy on sale or in bulk.

This guide was adapted from the Cornucopia Institute for buying soy products. For the full chart and report, go to www.cornucopia.org.[67]

Cornucopia Institute's SOY Guide (Modified Version)

Five Bean Rating
Eden Foods	Rhapsody Natural Foods	Twin Oaks
FarmSoy	Small Planet Tofu Shop	Unisoya
Green Cuisine		Vermont Soy

Four Bean Rating
Baby's Only Organic	Miso Master	Sunergia
Central Soyfoods	Nancy's	Tofurky
Fresh Tofu	Nasoya	Whole Soy
House Foods	Organic Valley	Wildwood
Lifeway	Soy Boy	Whole Foods (365)

Three Bean Rating
Harris Teeter	Pete's Tofu
O'Soy	Vitasoy

Two Bean Rating
Trader Joe's

One Bean Rating
Best Choice	Giant Eagle	Nature's Place
Full Circle	Greenwise	Wild Harvest
Laura Lynn	Pathmark	Weis Markets

No Bean Rating
Boca Burgers	Mori Nu Tofu	Soy Dream
Country Cream	Nature's Soy	Soya Deli
Earth's Best	Pacific Foods	Surata
Gardenburger	Pearl Soymilk	Westsoy
Helen's Kitchen	Sammi's Best	White Wave
Island Spring Tofu	Silk (Dean)	

Private Label
Archer Farms	Kirkland	Roundy's
Essensia	Nature's Promise	Shop Rite
Great Value	O Organics	Wegmans

6. Dairy

Family Farm

During the summer, my grandpa helped his grandma and grandpa on their farm in Thorp, Wisconsin by milking the cows twice a day. When the cows were not being milked, they would graze in the fields, warm themselves in the sun, and enjoy the summer breeze. Isn't this how cows are meant to live? These cows would live to be 20 plus years old. We were shocked to find out that only 1% of cows in the U.S. live like this, while 99% live on CAFO's.[68]

The cows on CAFO's live for about five years. Some are injected with bovine growth hormones (rBGH) to produce more milk and fed GMO grains and antibiotics to gain weight faster.[69] They spend their lives in a cycle of impregnation, birth, and milking, with a few breaks between pregnancies.[70]

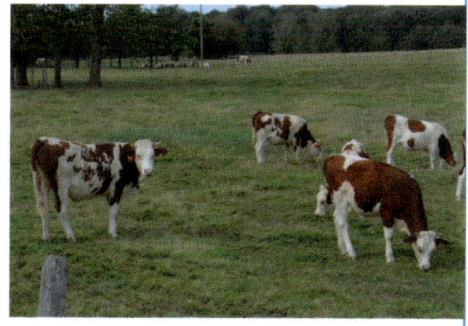

In 2007, the average cow in the dairy industry was forced to produce more than 20,000 pounds of milk in one year, twice the amount produced in my grandpa's day.[71] Mother Nature did not intend for cows to produce this much milk, and, as a result, the cows become very sick. When we drink milk from these sick cows, we are exposed to everything the cow ate and endured.

See meat section.

Questions to Ask

1. Did the cow eat grass, GMO grains, or organic grains?
2. Did the cow have antibiotics for illness or weight gain?
3. If organic, did the milk come from a CAFO or family farm?
4. Was the cow given growth hormones (rBGH)?
5. Did the cow live on a family farm or CAFO?

Follow the Cornucopia Institue's dairy guide! Ultra-pasteurization extends the shelf life of milk, but the heat destroys and kills nutrients and enzymes.[72]

Buy on sale, use coupons. Buy in bulk.

This guide was adapted from the Cornucopia Institute for buying dairy products.[73] For the full chart and report, go to www.cornucopia.org.

Cornucopia Institute's DAIRY Guide (Modified Version)
BUTTER / MARGARINE

What Should I Look For?

- From a family farm, through a CSA, farmers market, food co-op, or grocery store.
- Look for these labels: "100% grass-fed"
  "No growth hormones (rBGH)"
- Organic (no GMO's and no rBGH)
- Follow the Cornucopia Institute's chart, purchase brands rated "5" or "4," if not available, then buy brands rated "3" or "2."

What Should I Limit?

- Products rated "0," "1," or "Private Label"
- Growth hormones (rBGH)
- Margarines or spreads
- Artificial flavors, natural flavors, or additives

5 Cow Rating
Crystal Ball Farms (WI)
Fresh Breeze Organic Dairy (WA)
Kimball Brook Farm (VT)
Moo Maine's Own Organic (ME)
Organic Pastures Dairy Co. (CA)
PastureLand (MN)
Working Cow Dairy

4 Cow Rating
Hope Creamery (MN)
Westby Cooperative Creamery (WI)
Wisconsin Organics (WI)

2 Cow Rating
UNFI (Woodstock) (nationwide)

1 Cow Rating
Nature's Best (PA)

0 Cow Rating
Challenge Dairy Products (CA)
Grassland (WI)
Spring Hill Cheese/Petaluma Creamery (WI)

CHEESE

What Should I Look For?
- From a family farm, through a CSA, farmers market, or food co-op
- Look for these labels: "100% grass-fed"
  "No growth hormones (rBGH)"
- Organic (no GMO's and no rBGH)
- Follow the Cornucopia Institute's chart, purchase brands rated "5" or "4," if not available, then buy brands rated "3" or "2."

What Should I Limit?
- Products rated "0," "1," or "Private Label"
- Imitation cheese, artificial flavors, natural flavors or additives
- Growth hormones (rBGH) (not labeled if contains rBGH)

35

5 Cow Rating
Bridge View Dairy (PA)
Butternut Farms (NY)
Castle Rock Farms (WI)
Chase Hill Farm (MA)
Crystal Ball Farms (WI)
Hails Family Farm (PA)
Hawthorne Valley Farm (NY)
Lifeline Farm (MT)
Loleta Cheese (CA)
PastureLand (MN)
Thistle Hill Farm (VT)

4 Cow Rating
Cedar Grove Cheese (WI)
Cowgirl Creamery (CA)
Glanbia Foods (ID)
Green Field Farms (OH)
Kalona Supernatural (IA)
Organic Creamery (WI)
Sierra Nevada Cheese Co. (CA)
Westby Cooperative Creamery (WI)
Wisconsin Organics (WI)

1 Cow Rating
Nature's Best (CA)

0 Cow Rating
Back to Nature (Kraft) (IL)
Greenbank Farms/Stonefelt Cheese Co. (WA)
Rumiano Cheese Co. (CA)
Swissland (IN)
Wholesome Valley (FL)

COTTAGE CHEESE

What Should I Look For?

- From a family farm, through a CSA, farmers market, food co-op, or grocery store
- Look for these labels: "100% grass-fed"
  "No growth hormones (rBGH)"
- Organic (no GMO's and no rBGH)
- Follow the Cornucopia Institute's chart, purchase brands rated "5" or "4," if not available, then buy brands rated "3" or "2."

⚠ What Should I Limit?

- Products on Cornucopia Institute's chart rated a "1" or "0"
- Growth hormones (rBGH) (not labeled)

4 Cow Rating
Nancy's (OR)

CREAM CHEESE

What Should I Look For?

- From a family farm, through a CSA, farmers market, or food co-op
- Look for these labels: "No growth hormones (rBGH)"
- Organic (no GMO's and no rBGH)
- Follow the Cornucopia Institute's chart, purchase brands rated "5" or "4," if not available, then buy brands rated "3" or "2."

⚠ What Should I Limit?

- Products on Cornucopia Institute's chart rated a "1" or "0"
- Growth hormones (rBGH) (not labeled)

4 Cow Rating
Nancy's (OR)

ICE CREAM

What Should I Look For?

- Make your own.
- From a family farm, through a CSA, farmers market, food co-op, or grocery store
- Cream from grass-fed cows or rBGH-free milk
- Look for these labels: "No growth hormones (rBGH)."
- Organic (no GMO's and no rBGH)
- Follow the Cornucopia Institute's chart, purchase brands rated "5" or "4," if not available, then buy brands rated "3" or "2."

What Should I Limit?

- Products on Cornucopia Institute's chart rated a "1" or "0"
- Growth hormones (rBGH) (not labeled)
- Artificial or natural flavors, soy, powdered milk, or additives

5 Cow Rating
Cedar Summit Dairy (MN)
Crystal Ball Farm (WI)
Kimball Brook Farm (VT)

4 Cow Rating
Alden's Organic (OR)
Boulder Ice cream (CO)
Green and Black's (NJ)
Julie's (OR)
Natural Choice (CA)
Perry's Ice cream (NY)
Sibby Farm (WI)
Straus Family Creamery (CA)
Three Twins Organic (CA)
Wallaby Yogurt (CA)
Whole Foods (365)

3 Cow Rating
Boulder ice cream (CO)
Natural Choice (CA)

1 Cow Rating
Mr. Cookie Face (NJ)

The Weston A. Price Foundation recommends the following brands. For more brands and suggestions, go to www.westonaprice.org.[lxxiv]

Example Brands to Buy

Alden's organic ice cream
Ben & Jerry's vanilla ice cream
Copper Creek Farms raw goat ice cream
Grazin' Acres raw ice cream
Guernsey Dairy ice cream
Julie's organic ice cream
Kirkland Super Premium vanilla ice cream
Organicville vanilla and strawberry ice cream
Sibby's organic ice cream
Stonyfield Farm organic ice cream
Straus Family Creamery organic ice cream
Trader Joe's Super Premium French vanilla ice cream
Willow Run Dairy raw ice cream

MILK

What Should I Look For?

🐄 From a family farm, through a CSA, farmers market, food co-op, or grocery store.

🐄 Look for these labels: "No growth hormones (rBGH)"

🐄 Organic (no GMO's and no rBGH)

🐄 Follow the Cornucopia Institute's chart, purchase brands rated "5" or "4," if not available, then buy brands rated "3" or "2."

⚠ What Should I Limit?

🐄 Products on Cornucopia Institute's chart rated a "1" or "0"

🐄 Growth hormones (rBGH)

5 Cow Rating

Bridge View Dairy (PA)	Natural by Nature (PA)
Castle Rock Farms (WI)	New England Organic Creamery (MA)
Cedar Summit Dairy (MN)	Organic Acres (ID)
Chase Hill Farm (MA)	Organic Pastures Dairy Co. (CA)
Coonridge Dairy (goat) (NM)	Pride and Joy Dairy (OR)
Evans Farmhouse Creamery (NY)	Radiance Dairy (IA)
Crystal Ball Farms (WI)	Redwood Hill Farm/Creamery (CA)
Fresh Breeze Organic Dairy (WA)	Sandy River Farm (ME)
Hails Family Farm (cow and goat) (PA)	Sassy Cow Creamery (WI)
Hawthorne Valley Farm (NY)	St. John's Organic Farms (ID)
Kimball Brook Farm (VT)	Strafford Organic Creamery (VT)
Kimberton Hills (PA)	Traders Point Creamery (IN)
MOO Maine's Own Organic Milk (ME)	Working Cows Dairy (AL)

4 Cow Rating

Alpenrose Dairy (OR)	Scenic Central Co-op (WI)
Amish Country Farms (WI)	Stonyfield (NH)
Clover Organic Farms (CA	Straus Family Creamery (CA)
HyVee (IA)	Stremicks (CA)
Ingles Market (Harvest Farms) (SC)	Sunnyside Farms (CA)
Kalona Supernatural (IA)	Trickling Springs Creamery (PA)
Mom's organic market (VA)	Upstate Farms (NY)
Old Home (MN)	Wegmans Food Markets (NY)
Organic Valley (WI)	Whole Foods (365 organics)
Save Mart (CA)	Wisconsin's Organics (WI)

3 Cow Rating
Harris Teeter (South East)			Sky Top Farms (NY)

2 Cow Rating
Fairway (NY)				TESCO
Publix (SouthEast)			UNFI (Woodstock)
Stop & Shop (Natures Promise)		Wakefern/Shoprite

1 Cow Rating
Albertson's (Wild Harvest)		Nature's Basket (PA)
Assoc. Wholesale Grocers		Nature's Best (CA)
(Clearly Organic)			Our Family Organic (MN)
BJ's Wholesale Club			Price Choppers (Naturals)
Costco (Kirkland)			Roundy's (WI)
Earth Fare (NC)				Safeway (O - Organics)
Giant (Natures Promise)			Sprouts/Henry Market (CA)
Great Value (Wal-mart)			Stew Leonard's (NY)
HEB/Central Market			Target (Archer Farms)
Kroger (Simple Truth)			Topco (Full Circle)
Lund's and Byerly's (MN)		Trader Joe's
Meijer, Inc. (MI)			Western Family Foods (OR)
Meijer's Organic (MI)			Winn-Dixie (FL)

0 Cow Rating
Aurora Organic Dairy			Humboldt Creamery
Borden Dairy (Dean)			Kemp's Dairy (dean)
Champlain Valley Dairy (NY)		Mother's Choice (GA)
Good Heart Organics (CA)		Natural Prairie (TX)
Dean and Horizon (Dean)			Shamrock Farms

YOGURT

What Should I Look For?

- Make your own.
- From a family farm, through a CSA, farmers market, food co-op, or grocery store
- Organic (no GMO's and no rBGH)
- Look for these labels: "Grass-fed milk"
  "No growth hormones (rBGH)"
- Plain, whole fat, add your own fruit
- Follow the Cornucopia Institute's chart, purchase brands rated **"5" or "4,"** if not available, then buy brands rated **"3" or "2."**

What Should I Limit?

- Products on Cornucopia Institute's chart rated a "1" or "0"
- Growth hormones, artificial flavors, natural flavors, or additives

5 Cow Rating

Butterworks Farm	Maple Hill Creamery
Cedar Summit Dairy	Radiance Dairy
Crystal Ball Farms	Redwood Hill Farm and Creamery
Hails Family Farm	Seven Stars
Hawthorne Valley Farm	Traders Point Creamery (IN)

4 Cow Rating

Cascade Fresh	Stonyfield
(Kalona Organics)	Straus Family Creamery
Cultural Revolution	Wallaby
Nancy's	

1 Cow Rating

Happy Baby
White Mountain Foods

7. Eggs

Local   Family Farm   Local

One of my good friends raises chickens on her farm in North Hampton, New Hampshire. When my children visited her, their job was to feed the chickens and gather their eggs. They would collect the kitchen scraps and toss them to the chickens. The chickens would also wander through the grass, using their beaks to eat bugs, worms, and anything else they could get their beaks into. My friend recollected her wonder at how a beautiful egg, full of nutrients, was delivered every morning. She said the health of the egg was determined by the yolk, not the color of the shell. Each golden yolk was full of vitamins and nutrients.

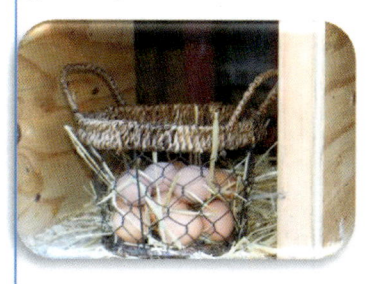

Unfortunately, the majority of chickens do not lay their eggs on family farms, but in large metal barns. These chickens are kept in very small cages, for about two years.[75] The cages are stacked on top of one another. This environment causes a great deal of stress for the chickens.[76] They are fed GMO corn and antibiotics. Antibiotics are used to keep them alive, because this environment makes them very, very sick. These cages, by the way, are banned in the European Union."[77]

The industry wants to meet the "market demand." In 2007, these metal barns made it possible for 280 million hens to lay 77.3 billion eggs.[78] This is feasible by artificially inducing the chickens. In addition, to shock their bodies into another egg-laying cycle when production declines, hens are sometimes starved and denied any food for up to two weeks.[79] The birds are not able to roam outside for exercise, enjoy the sunshine, or eat bugs and worms. As a result, these eggs have a pale yolk surrounded by a thin shell. Studies have shown that diet, lack of sunlight, and no exercise have a great impact on the quality of the eggs produced.

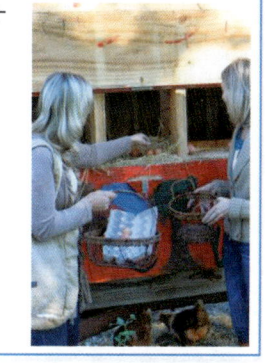

> The eggs from my friend's farm are now considered a specialty item sought out by many and paid for at a higher price. These eggs are usually not sold in the grocery store, but rather directly from the farm at farmers markets, food co-ops, and through Community Supported Agriculture (CSA).

> A pale yolk means the chicken lived in crowded conditions and lacked a good diet. A darker, golden yellow yolk means the chicken lived outdoors and ate a good diet. According to studies, chickens spending time outside and eating a diet they are meant to eat, produce eggs with omega-3 fatty acids, beta carotene, and vitamins A, D, and E, unlike eggs from CAFO chicken eggs.[80]

Important Terms to Know

- Free-range and pasture-raised are not regulated.[81,82]
- Cage-free: chickens are not kept in cages, but are kept inside metal barns and fed an unhealthy diet.
- USDA certified organic: chickens are fed organic, non-GMO feed, without pesticides and antibiotics.[83] They are not in cages, but may still be in metal barns.
- No hormones given: hormones are not allowed in chickens, so this product is not better than another, it's only a marketing term.
- The only national grocery store chain to have banned the sale of eggs from caged hens is Whole Foods.[84]
- The only restaurant chain to promise to ban them from their supply chain is Burger King (by 2017).[85]
- Small cages (battery cages) will be illegal in California, in 2015, and in Michigan, in 2019.[86]

Questions to Ask

1. Is the chicken from a CAFO or family farm?
2. Was the chicken able to be outdoors for exercise?
3. Does the poultry contain dyes, additives, or natural flavors?
4. What did the chicken eat?
5. Did the chicken live in a cage in a metal building or was it in a chicken coop, spending most of its time outside?
6. Was the chicken fed antibiotics for weight gain or for illness?

What Should I Look For?
- Directly from a family farm, through a CSA, farmers market, or food co-op
- Follow the Cornucopia Institute's chart for the best choices. Buy brands rated "5" or "4," if not available, then "3" or "2."

What Should I Limit?
- Products on this chart rated a "0," "1," or private label
- Natural, free-range, cage-free, or pasteurized shell eggs

Buy directly from the farm, farm fresh eggs are only $0.37- per egg!

To get the most from your egg dollars, buy them direclty from the farmer.

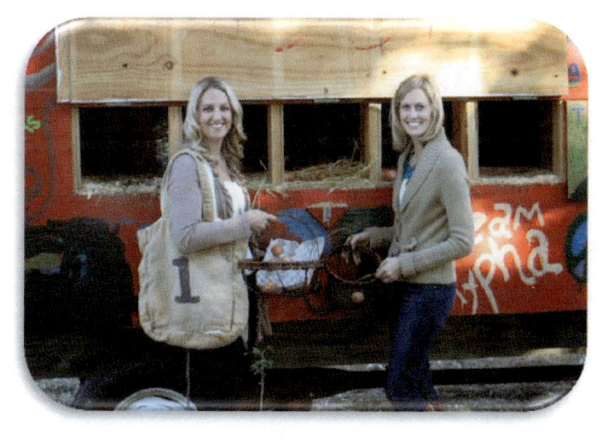

This guide was adapted from the Cornucopia Institute for buying egg products.[87] For the full chart and report, go to www.cornucopia.org.

Cornucopia Institute's EGG Guide (Modified Version)

5 Egg Rating

Alexandre Kids	Mosel Eggs
Amsterdam Organics	Neversink Farm
Bee Heaven Farm	Old Friends Farm
Burroughs Family Farms Eggs	One Drop Farm
Cleary Family Farm	Organic Pastures
Common Good Farm	Phoenix Egg Farm
Coon Creek	PNS Farms
Doolittle Farm	River Berry Farm
Dreamfarm	Schultz Eggs
First Frost Farm	Shenandoah Family
Green Hills Harvest	Skagit River Ranch
Green Pastures Poultry	St. John Family Farm
Handsome Brook Farm	Stony Brook Valley
Happy Town Farm	Trout Lake Abbey
Highfields Farm	Turtle Ledge Farm
Kingbird Farm	Village Farm
Krause Farm	Vital Farms
Lazy 69 Ranch	WAG Eggs
Mission Mountain	Whispering Spruce
Misty Meadows Farm	World's Best Eggs
Morning Sun Farm	

4 Egg Rating

B Dabler	Milo's Organic	New Century
Hi Q Organic	Misera Family Farm	

3 Egg Rating

Born Free	Giving Nature	Pete & Gerry's
Clover Organic Farms	Green Field Farms	Stiebrs Farms
Egg Innovations	Nature's Yoke	Wilcox Farms
Farmers' Hen House	Organic Valley	

2 Egg Rating

Sauder's	The Country Hen

1 Egg Rating

Abbotsford
Barnstar Family Farms
Big Island Poultry
Bob LaPlace
Canoe Creek
Chino Valley Ranchers
Circle JD Ranch
Clark Summit Farm
Eggland's Best
Eggology
Eight Mile Creek Farm
Farmer's Harvest
Flying Dutchman Farm
Garden Valley
Giroux Poultry Farm
Glaum Egg Ranch
Herbruck Poultry Ranch
Hillanddale Farms
Horizon Organic
Hotz Farms
Judy's Family Farm
Land O'Lakes
Nest Fresh Eggs
Oakdell
Organic Acres
Persimmon Pond
Pine Belt Eggs
Reading Creek Ranch
Redhill Farms
Sparboe
Tree of Life
Vega Farms

Private Label

Archer Farms
Cadia
Central Market
Country Creek
Crack a Smile
Full Circle
Great Value
Green Way
Kirkland Signature
Lucerne Foods
Lunds
Meijer Organics
Natural Directions
Natural Selections
Naturally Preferred
Nature's Basket
Nature's Place
Nature's Promise
O Organic
Price Chopper Naturals
Publix
Roundy's Organics
Trader Joe's
United Egg Producers
Wegman's
Whole Foods (365)
Wild Harvest

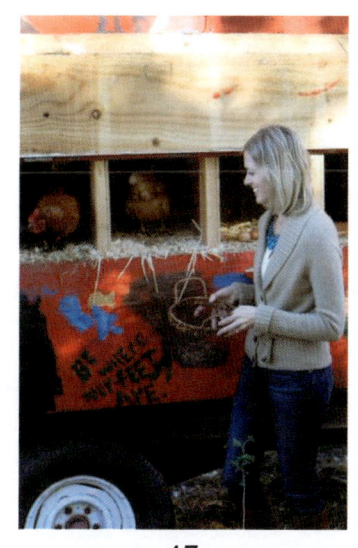

8. In the Aisles

Bake Organic Bake

Families used to spend more time in the kitchen cooking and baking. Remember when Mom or Grandma made cookies, bread, and spaghetti sauce from scratch? Foods like pancake mix, chicken nuggets, instant macaroni and cheese, and slice-and-bake cookies were not available, and bread was baked at home or purchased from a bakery or specialty shop. Today, we live in a grab-and-go society. We are busier than ever with work, school, sports, and other extracurricular activities, leaving less time for preparing good, high-quality, healthy meals. We just don't have time to spend hours in the kitchen kneading bread dough or stewing tomatoes. Instead, we opt for a quick, seemingly nutritious, meal instead.

The FDA requires nutritional information on all packaged foods. To a certain degree, consumers have been trained to read labels. But if you are like most people, you only look at the calories and fat grams. Some, more health-conscious individuals, might look at the sodium levels and sugar grams, and others may check to see if the product contains high-fructose corn syrup. The problem, however, is that most consumers are looking at the wrong part of the label! As consumers, we need to scrutinize the ingredient list. Michael Pollan, American author and food activist, writes in his work, *Food Rules: Eater's Manual,* about the importance of eating foods with no more than five ingredients.[88] He also writes, "Avoid food products containing ingredients that a third-grader cannot pronounce!"[89] In the end, what you are actually putting in your mouth, is right in the ingredient list, and not on the nutritional label.

Some say that there are so many preservatives in our food that our bodies will long be preserved after our death. The five-ingredient rule is a great, easy directive to remember. The problem with most prepackaged foods is that they are filled with additives. These foods contain preservatives and other chemicals used solely to enhance the shelf life, flavor, or appearance of the food. These chemicals are not making you healthy. On the contrary, many of these foods contain high-fructose corn syrup, trans fats, and GMO ingredients, all of which contribute to rapid weight gain, increased risk for cancers, headaches, and stomachaches, among other ailments.[90][91][92] Take a bag of popular brand crackers, for example. They are low in calories, low in overall fat, but contain the following chemicals and preservatives: Thiamine Mononitrate (artificially created B-1 vitamin), high-fructose corn syrup, soybean oil (another GMO that contains trans fats), cotton seed oil (another trans fat), soy lecithin (a GMO food preservative), natural flavor (a laboratory-made cracker flavor REALLY!), and defatted wheat germ (a texture and flavor enhancer that requires hexane and petroleum to break it down so it is usable in foods). A cracker should consist of just flour, water, and salt, and, perhaps, an herb or two! *The closer a food is to its natural state, or source, the better it is for you.* Every time a food is processed, vital nutrients are lost. Eating foods as they are purely found in nature, such as fresh vegetables, fruits, pure olive oil, butter, raw honey, raw sugar, and whole grains is a smart choice!

Healthy food doesn't have to take hours to prepare, you just have to know what and what not to choose. It is true that in today's grab-and-go society, we have less time for preparing high quality, healthy meals made from scratch. There are, however, plenty of families who prioritize their time to cook and bake. The book, *Make the Bread, Buy the Butter*, by Jennifer Reese, is a great place to start. The author also lets you know how much money you'll save! You must decide what is important to you. And, if you are reading this book, you are definitely on the right track!!

Bake! Read *Make the Bread, Buy the Butter* by Jennifer Reese

Buy on sale. Use coupons. Buy in bulk. Bake!

Questions to Ask

1. Does this product contain partially hydrogenated oils?
2. Does this product contain fiber?
3. Does this product contain GMO's?
4. Does this product contain a long list of ingredients?
5. Does this product contain corn ingredients?
6. Does this product contain trans-fat?
7. Does this product contain sugar?

Baby Foods

What Should I Look For?
- Make your own
- Organic
- Glass jars or BPA-free plastic containers

What Should I Limit?
- DHA added from DHA made in a lab
- BPA plastic containers

This guide was adapted from the Cornucopia Institute.[93] For the full chart and report, go to www.cornucopia.org.

Example Brands to Buy

Earth's Best	Petite Palate	Sweet Pea Baby Food
Ella's Kitchen	Plum Organics	Yummy Spoonfuls
Gerber organic	Revolution Foods	Happy Baby (products, except cereal)
Healthy Times	Sprout Organics	
Jack's Harvest	Square One	
Organic Baby	Stonyfield Farms	

Baking Powder

What Should I Look For?
- Aluminum-free baking powder

What Should I Limit?
- Aluminum baking powder

The Weston A. Price Foundation recommends the following brands. For more brands and suggestions, go to www.westonaprice.org.[94]

Example Brands to Buy *(aluminum-free)*
- Bob's Red Mill aluminum-free baking powder
- Frontier aluminum-free baking powder
- Mary Jane's Farm aluminum-free baking powder
- Rumford aluminum-free baking powder

Breads

What Should I Look For?
- Bake it in your bread machine with organic whole grain flour.
- Organic breads from your local bakery or famers market.
- Sourdough or sprouted breads

What Should I Limit?
- Additives, soy flour, or partially hydrogenated vegetable oils
- Gluten
- Whole grain is better than multigrain

The Weston A. Price Foundation recommends the following brands. For more brands and suggestions, go to www.westonaprice.org.[95]

Example Brands to Buy
Acme Bakery sour dough rye acme bakery pain au levain
Bonus Vivius rye/spelt bread
Grindstone Bakery bread
Hawthorne Valley Sourdough rye
Le Pain Quotidien Leavin bread
Miller's Organic Farm breads
Mountain Eagle Bakery breads
Orchard Hills Breadworks breads
Pacific Bakery breads
Pleasanton Brick Oven Bakery
Serenity Farm sourdough breads
Trader Joe's Organic Flourless Sprouted 7-Grain Bread
Vermont Bread Company Baldwin Hill sourdough rye bread
Vital Vittles sourdough rye and Russian sourdough
Whole Foods organic whole wheat sourdough bread
Whole Foods pain de campaigne (sourdough)

Cake Mix

What Should I Look For?
- Organic
- Make your own

⚠ What Should I Limit?
- Soy flour or bleached white flour
- Long, complicated ingredient list

Candy and Chocolate

What Should I Look For?
- Organic
- Fair trade
- 70% or more dark chocolate
- The ingredient list should state organic cane sugar, evaporated cane juice, or organic sugar

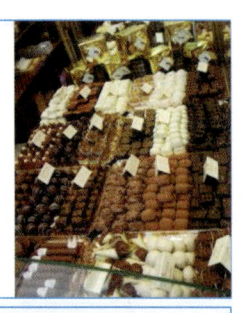

⚠ What Should I Limit?
- Partially hydrogenated oils, soy lecithin, or corn syrup

The Non-GMO project has verified that these brands do not contain GMO's. For more brands and suggestions, go to www.nongmoproject.org.[96]

Example Brands to Buy
Alter Eco (all brands)
Amella Vegan Coconut Almond Caramels
Amella Vegan Gray Sea Salt Caramels
Endangered Species dark chocolate (not milk chocolate)
Essential Living Foods Chocolate Covered Cacao Nibs
Essential Living Foods Raw Decadence Dark Chocolate Bar
Go Raw 100% Organic Real Live Chocolate Mint
Go Raw 100% Organic Real Live Chocolate Mint
Go Raw 100% Organic Real Live Chocolate Orange
Go Raw 100% Organic Real Live Chocolate Original
Heavenly Organics Honey Pattie Chocolate Almond

Heavenly Organics Honey Pattie Chocolate Coconut
Heavenly Organics Honey Pattie Chocolate Ginger
Heavenly Organics Honey Pattie Chocolate Mint
Heavenly Organics Honey Pattie Chocolate Pomegranate
Kur Organic Superfood Delights Dark Chocolate Mint
Multiple Organics Organic Cocoa Nibs
Multiple Organics Organic Dark Chocolate Drops
Multiple Organics Organic Fair Trade Chocolate Covered Cocoa Nibs
NibMor Daily Dose of Dark
NibMor Daily Dose of Dark 72% mint & nibs
NibMor Dark Chocolate Original
NibMor Dark Chocolate with Almonds
NibMor Dark Chocolate with Brown Rice Crispy
NibMor Dark Chocolate with Cacao Nibs Extreme
NibMor Dark Chocolate with Mint + Nibs
Righteously Raw (all brands) (gluten free, top 8 allergen free)
Sun Cups (all brands) (nut free, gluten free)
Theo (all brands except milk chocolate)
Two Moms in the Raw Gluten-Free Almond Butter Cacao Truffle
Vega Maca Chocolate

Cereal

What Should I Look For?

Follow the Cornucopia Institute's chart, buy brands rated a "5" or "4," if not available, then "3" or "2"

What Should I Limit?

Products rated "1" on the Cornucopia Institute's chart
Products labeled "Natural"

> This guide was adapted from the Cornucopia Institute for buying cereal.[97] For the full chart and report, go to www.cornucopia.org.

Cornucopia Institute CEREAL Guide (Modified Version)

5 Grain Rating
Ambrosial	Grandy Oats	Lydia's Organics
Country Choice	Great River	Nature's Path
Organic	Organic Milling	Tierra Farm
Farm to Table	Kaia	Two Moms
Go Raw	Laughing Giraffe	In the Raw

4 Grain Rating
Eco-Planet	Food for Life	Green Barn
Erewhon	Grawnola	Organics

3 Grain Rating
Annie's	Grizzlie's Brand	Skinners
Homegrown	New England	Stark Sisters
Cascadian Farm	Naturals	Granola
Cream of the West	Ruth's Hemp Foods	Uncle Sam
Weetabix		

2 Grain Rating
Alpen	Dorset Cereal	Sweet Home Farm
Arrowhead Mills	Health Valley	
Back to Nature	Mother's	
Bob's Red Mill	Peace Cereal	

1 Grain Rating
Bakery on Main	General Mills	Post Natural
Barbara's Bakery	Mom's Best	Three Sisters
Bear Naked	Nutritious Living	Udi's Granola
Kashi	OLA!	

Chips

What Should I Look For?
- Cooked in lard, or coconut, olive, or peanut oil

What Should I Limit?
- Partially hydrogenated vegetable oil

The Weston A. Price Foundation recommends the following brands. For more brands and suggestions, go to www.westonaprice.org.[98]

Example Brands to Buy

Abuelita's tortilla chips (in peanut oil)

Aimee's Livin' Magic onion chips

Aimee's Livin' Magic zucchini chips

Boulder Canyon olive oil potato chips

Chef Garcia tortilla chips (in peanut oil)

Clancy's olive oil potato chips

Danielle chips (except those containing sugar)

Food Should Taste Good yellow corn tortilla chips

Freeland Foods Go Raw spirulina super chips

Good Health avocado oil potato chips (sea salt and barbeque)

Good Health olive oil potato chips

Good potato chips (in lard)

Grandma Utz's potato chips (in lard)

Honest potato chips (in coconut oil)

Inka cassava or mixed chips

Inka original corn or sweet potato

Inka original or sweet plantain

Koyo organic brown rice chips

Live Superfoods spirulina super chips

Maine Coast sea chips

Meadow Ridge Farm potato chips (in pastured lard)

Nana's Cocina tortilla chips (in peanut oil)

The Raw Food World coconut crisps

The Raw Food World onion crisps

The Raw Food World spirulina super chips

The Raw Food World zucchini chips

Trader Joe's Red Bliss potato chips (in olive oil)

Utz Kettle Classics potato chips (in peanut oil)

Utz organic corn tortilla chips

Way Better tortilla chips

Coconut

What Should I Look For?
- Buy brands that have these words on the label:
  - Water, milk, cream extracted from fresh coconuts
  - Whole canned coconut milk without additives
  - Canned coconut cream without additives
  - Coconut vinegar
- BPA-free cans

What Should I Limit?
- "Lite" coconut milk or sweetened coconut meat
- Preservatives
- Cans lined with BPA

The Weston A. Price Foundation recommends the following brands. For more brands and suggestions, go to www.westonaprice.org.[99]

Example Brands to Buy
A Taste of Thai whole coconut milk
Glaser Organic Farms fresh organic coconut water
Good Stuff by Mom & Me raw coconut vinegar
Living Tree coconut crème
Living Tree coconut vinegar
Native Forest organic whole coconut milk
Natural Value coconut milk
So Delicious coconut milk
Thai Kitchen organic whole coconut milk
Tropical Traditions coconut crème concentrate

Cookies

What Should I Look For?
- Make your own
- Organic

What Should I Limit?
- Soy protein isolate
- High-fructose corn syrup and partially hydrogenated oil

The Weston A. Price Foundation recommends the following brands. For more brands and suggestions, go to www.westonaprice.org.[100]

Example Brands to Buy
Alive and Radiant Foods raweo cookies and lemon swirls
Beccaroons macaroons
Berkshire Mountain Bakery ginger molasses cookies
Diviana Alchemy lucuma cookie bites
Freeland Foods Go Raw super cookies (except chocolate)
Sweetwater Baking Co. wholesome cookies
The Raw Food World lucuma cookie bites
The Raw Food World raweo coolies, lemon swirls, original super cookies, ginger snaps, lemon pie coco-roons
Ultimate Superfoods lucuma cookie bites

Crackers

What Should I Look For?
- Organic
- Ground whole grain flour, sourdough, or sprouted
- Made with wheat, rice or oats

What Should I Limit?
- Additives
- Partially hydrogenated oils, soy flour, and gluten

The Weston A. Price Foundation recommends the following brands. For more brands and suggestions, go to www.westonaprice.org.[101]

Example Brands to Buy
Aimee's Livin' Magic 'kraut chia crackers
Aimee's Livin' Magic apple cinnamon snappers
Aimee's Livin' Magic kimchi crackers
It's Alive! sprouted sauerkraut and kimchi crackers
Mary's Gone Crackers (gluten-free)
Natural Zing sprouted sauerkraut and kimchi crackers
RawGuru sprouted sauerkraut crackers
Ry Krisp light rye crackers
The Raw Food World curry, 'kraut chia crackers
The Raw Food World kimchi crackers
Wasa light rye crispbread

Flour

What Should I Look For?
- Organic
- Unbleached white flour

⚠ What Should I Limit?
- Bleached white flour or soy flour

The Weston A. Price Foundation recommends the following brands. For more brands and suggestions, go to www.westonaprice.org.[102]

Example Brands to Buy
Bob's Red Mill unbleached white flour
King Arthur organic unbleached white flour

Frozen Dinners

We don't recommend frozen dinners. If you buy them, go organic.

Granola and Nutrition Bars

What Should I Look For?
- Make your own
- Organic
- Follow the guide below, have the bars colored in **green** and **purple**.

⚠ What Should I Limit?
- Hexane (soy protein isolate) or high-fructose corn syrup
- Have the bars colored **red** in moderation.

This guide was adapted from the Cornucopia Institute for buying nutrition bars.[103] For the full chart and research report, go to www.cornucopia.org.

Cornucopia Institute's NUTRION BAR Guide (Modified Version)

These brands are Organic and do NOT have soy protein isolate

- Alpsnack (all bars)
- Amazing Grass (green superfood)
- Bear Fruit (all bars)
- Bumble Bar (all bars)
- Clif Nectar (nectar bars)
- Garden of Life (living food bars)
- Genisoy (organic bars)
- Hammer (all bars)
- Honey Stinger (protein bars)
- Nutiva (all bars)
- Nature's Path (optimum bars)
- Organic Food Bar (all bars)
- Potent Foods (Potent Life Bars)
- Pure (pure bars)
- Raw Revolution (all bars)
- Wild Bar (all bars)
- Zen Organic Foods (all bars)

Non-Organic brands, but do NOT contain soy protein isolate

- Clif "C" Bar (70% of ingredients are organic)
- Odwalla (original bars, superfood bars, chewy nut bars)
- Kind Plus (antioxidants bars)
- SoyJoy (all bars)
- Vega (Vega Whole Food bars)

Non-Organic, but contain soy protein isolate

- Balance Bar (Original, Bare, Gold and Carbwell Bars)
- Can Do Kid (all bars)
- Clif Bar (all Clif bars)
- Clif Builder's Bar (all Builder's bars)
- Clif Mojo Bar (all Mojo bars)
- Genisoy (Non-Organic Bars and Ultra and Protein Crunch bars)
- Greens Plus (energy bars)
- Honey Stinger (energy bars)
- Kind Plus (protein bars)
- Luna Bar (all bars)
- Luna Protein Bar (all bars)
- NuGo (non-organic bars)
- Odwalla (protein bars)
- Power Bar (Harvest and Nut Naturals bars) Pria Bar (all bars)
- Promax (Promax and Promax 70 bars)
- Pure Protein (all bars)
- Think (Think Thin Protein and Crunch bars)
- Whole Foods 365 (Super Greens bar)
- Zone Perfect (Zone Perfect and Fruitified bars)

Honey

What Should I Look For?
- Labels that say: "Raw," "Unfiltered," or "Pure"
- Honey in a glass container

What Should I Limit?
- Honey with corn syrup (may contain corn syrup if it doesn't state raw, unfiltered, or pure on bottle)
- In a plastic bottle

Jam

What Should I Look For?
- Farmers market, local health food store, CSA, or grocery store
- Organic or cane sugar

What Should I Limit?
- High-fructose corn syrup, artificial sweeteners, and corn syrup

The Weston A. Price Foundation recommends the following brands. For more brands and suggestions, go to www.westonaprice.org.[104]

Example Brands to Buy
Bionaturae fruit spreads
Colorado Mountain jams
Copper Creek Farms jams, jellies, and preserves
Crofter's organic fruit spreads
Eden fruit butters
Fiordifrutta fruit spreads
Grazin' Acres jams and apple butter
Hoskins Berry Farm fruit spreads
Kahiltna Birchworks wild mixed berry fruit spread
Miller's Biodiversity Farm apple butter
Miller's Organic Farm apple butter
Selina Naturally fruit spreads

Muffins

What Should I Look For?
- Make your own
- Made with whole grain flour and cane sugar

⚠ What Should I Limit?
- Partially hydrogenated vegetable oil or high-fructose corn syrup
- Long, complicated ingredient list

Oils

What Should I Look For?
- Organic extra virgin olive oil (unfiltered)
- Virgin coconut oil and unrefined palm oil
- Cold pressed oils: sesame, sunflower, peanut, flax, and high oleic safflower oil

⚠ What Should I Limit? (These oils are heavily processed, so little of the original oil is left.)
- Non-organic oils: vegetable, canola, cottonseed, soy, corn, hemp, and grapeseed.
- Margarines and partially-hydrogenated vegetable shortening
- Epichlorophydrin (in refined oils)

The Weston A. Price Foundation recommends the following brands. For more brands and suggestions, go to www.westonaprice.org.[105]

Example Brands to Buy
Apollo extra virgin olive oil
Bariani organic extra virgin olive oil
Bionaturae organic extra virgin olive oil
Eden extra virgin olive and organic unrefined sesame oils
Equal Exchange organic extra virgin olive oil
Garden of Life virgin coconut oil
Kirkland extra virgin olive oil
Napa Valley Naturals organic extra virgin olive oil

Radiant Life organic extra virgin olive oil
Spectrum extra virgin olive oil
Spectrum organic extra virgin unfiltered olive oil
Spectrum organic palm shortening
Spectrum unrefined sesame oils
Spectrum virgin coconut oil
Trader Joe's organic extra virgin olive oil
Trader Joe's organic virgin coconut oil

*NOTE: Oils have different cooking points. Olive oil has a low cooking point, so cooking with it releases toxins into foods. Add olive oil at the end or use it as dipping oil. Coconut oil is better for frying since it can withstand high heat.

Pancake Mix

What Should I Look For?
- Organic
- Make your own

What Should I Limit?
- Non-organic

Example Brands to Buy

| 1-2-3 Gluten Free | Arrowhead Mills | Bob Red Mill |

Pasta

What Should I Look For?
- Make it at home or buy it at the farmers market.
- Organic

What Should I Limit?
- High-fructose corn syrup

Example Brands to Buy

| Bionaturae | DeBoles | DeLallo |

Pasta Sauce

What Should I Look For?
- Make your own (olive oil, crushed tomatoes, and spices)
- Organic
- Glass jar or BPA-free can

What Should I Limit?
- High-fructose corn syrup and partially hydrogenated oils

Example Brands to Buy

Bionaturae	Lucini	Eden
DeLallo	Pomi	Secret Recipe

Peanut Butter and Nut Butter

What Should I Look For?
- Make it at home (peanuts, peanut oil, salt).
- Organic or cane sugar

What Should I Limit?
- High-fructose corn syrup
- Sugar

Example Brands to Buy

Artisana	Justin's
I.M. Health SoyNut Butters	Maranatha Nut Butters

Popcorn

What Should I Look For?
- Make at home in an Air Pop machine or in a pan on the stove
- Corn from a farmers market

⚠ What Should I Limit?
- Microwave popcorn

Example Brands to Buy
Eden   Trader Joe's organic popcorn
Quinn popcorn

Seeds

What Should I Look For?
- Companies that have signed the Safe Seed Pledge

⚠ What Should I Limit?
- Seeds you have not researched.

Example Brands to Buy

Baker Creek Hierloom Seeds	Seeds of Change
Botanical Interests	Seeds Savers Exchange
Burpee Seeds and Plants	Southern Exposure Seed Exchange
Fedco Seeds	
Ferry-Morse Seed Company	Territorial Seed Company
High Mowing Seeds	The Cook's Garden
Johnny's Selected Seeds	
Nichols Garden Nursery	
Peaceful Valley Farm & Garden Supply	

Soups

What Should I Look For?
- Make homemade soups.
- Cans labeled "BPA free"

What Should I Limit?
- Bouillon cubes
- Non-organic

Example Brands to Buy
Amy's canned soups
Bar Harbor
Chesapeake Gardens soups

Sugar and Sweeteners

What Should I Look For?
- Local (in the United States)
- Organic sugar or organic pure cane sugar
- Organic stevia powder or organic stevia leaves
- 100% organic cane sugar or organic evaporated cane juice
- Organic: sucanat, maple sugar, date sugar, dehydrated sugar cane juice, coconut palm sugar, malt sugar, or sorghum syrup

What Should I Limit?
- Agave, fructose, high-fructose corn syrup, white sugar, sucralose, and Aspartame
- Beet sugar, labeled as "sugar" on ingredient list

The Weston A. Price Foundation recommends the following brands.[106] For more brands and suggestions, go to www.westonaprice.org.

Example Brands to Buy
Big Tree Farms organic coconut palm sugar
Branon organic sugar
Coconut Secret raw coconut crystal, coconut nectar
Coombs sugar
Divine Organics coconut sugar
Essential Living Foods green stevia powder
Essential Living Foods organic coconut sugar
Frontier green stevia powder
Glaser Organic Farms date sugar
Grazin' Acres coconut sugar
Heavenly Sugar
Live Superfoods organic coconut palm sugar
Living Tree coconut crystals
Living tree date sugar
Madhava organic blonde coconut crystals
Maple Hill Farm sugar
Mascavo organic sugar
Mestia raw blonde coconut sugar
Mother Linda's maple sugar
Mountian Rose Herbs stevia leaves and green powder
Muscovado sugar
Natural Zing green stevia powder
Natural Zing palm sugar
Nature's Blessings organic coconut sugar
Navitas Naturals green stevia powder
Navitas Naturals organic palm sugar
Nuts Online Organic palm sugar
Pangaia organic coconut sugar
Rapadura
RawGuru palm sugar
Selina Naturally coconut crystals
Shiloh Farms maple sugar and date sugar
Stannard Farm sugar
Sucanat
Sweet Tree organic palm sugars
The Raw Food World coconut sugar
Ultimate Superfoods organic palm sugar
Wholesome Sweeteners organic coconut palm sugar
Wilderness Family Naturals coconut sugar

Sugar 101

Note: the brands in this sugar section are brands commonly found on the shelf at the grocery store. For brands we recommend see page 67.

1. Sugars Found in the Fields

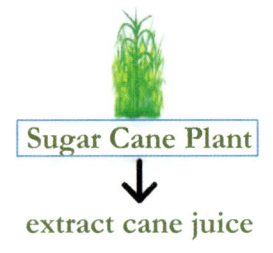

Sugar Cane Plant
↓
extract cane juice

evaporate, dehydrate, or boil down
↓
Cane Sugar
(if label says organic pure cane sugar, no GMO's)
(Brands: Florida Crystals, Wholesome Sweeteners, Rapunzel)

boil down
↓
Sucanat
(brown color because it contains molasses)
(may substitute for brown sugar)
(if label says organic pure cane sugar or organic cane sugar, no GMO's)
(Brands: Rapadura/Panela, Sugar Cane Naturals, Wholesome Sweeteners)

wash, remove molasses
↓
Raw Sugar
(substitute for brown sugar)
(if label says organic pure cane sugar or organic cane sugar, no GMO's)
(Brands: Organic Sugar in the Raw, Turbinado)

2. More Sugars Found in the Field

Date Sugar
(healthier than brown sugar, vitamins and nutrients intact)
(coarse, ground up dates or use date sugar for toppings on yogurt, ice cream, granola, cobblers, etc.)
(Brands: Bob's Red Mill, Now Foods)

Stevia
(healthier than brown sugar, vitamins/nutrients intact)
(Brands: Stevia, Rebaudiana)

Modified Sweeteners	Organic?	Brands	Miscellaneous
Agave nectar	Most are not organic and majority are highly processed with additives	Blue Agave Madhava Organic Raw	<u>Found In</u> Chocolate Ice cream Ketchup Nutrition bars
Stevia	Some are organic and some certified organic stevia is highly processed with added ingredients	Pure Via Rebaudiana Stevia Truvia	Grow a plant or buy pure dried leaves
Sucralose	No	Cuckren Nevella Splenda SucraPlus Candys Sukrana	320-1000x sweeter than sugar

Non-Sugar Sweeteners	Brands	Miscellaneous
Barley Malt Syrup	Eden Foods Organic King Arthur Organic	Baking, cooking, beer; malty flavor
Black Strap Molasses	Organic Molasses Wholesome Sweeteners	Used for baking, strong flavor
Brown Rice Syrup	Great Eastern Sun Sweet Cane Sweet Cloud Sweet Dreams Tropical Traditions Lunberg Farm	May have high arsenic levels
Maple Syrup	NOW Foods Shady Maple Farms	Used for pancakes, French toast, baking
Sorghum Syrup	Look for it at family farms	Mistaken for molasses (sorghum molasses)

3. Sugars made in the lab

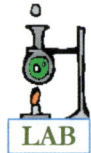

LAB

(designed to become resistance to glyphosate (herbicide)

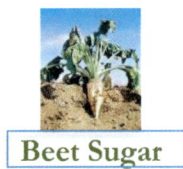

↓

Beet Sugar

(95% of crops in U.S. are GMO)
(if label says sugar, it is GMO)
(Brands: American Crystal Sugar Co.)

Dextrose

(GMO corn)

Artificial Sweeteners (GMO)	Brands
Aspartame	NutraSweet, Equal, Spoonful, EqualMeasure, AminoSweet
High-fructose corn syrup	Corn sweetener, corn syrup, corn sugar
Neotame	Sweetos (used in cattle feed)
Saccharin	Sweet & Low, Sugar twin

Syrup

What Should I Look For?
- Farmers market, local health food store, CSA, or grocery store
- 100% pure organic maple syrup

What Should I Limit?
- High-fructose corn syrup and artificial flavors
- Syrup with lard (added to reduce foaming)

The Weston A. Price Foundation recommends the following brands.[107] For more brands and suggestions, go to www.westonaprice.org.

Example Brands to Buy

Back Creek
Beech Road Moo Juicing Farm organic
Branon organic
Buck Mountain
Coombs
Copper Creek Farms
Eagle's Sugar Camp
Eden organic barley malt and sorghum
Grazin'Acres maple and sorghum
Highland Sugarworks organic
Kahiltna Birchworks birch
Kickapoo Gold
Living Tree

Maple Hill Farm
Maple Syrup Producers' Cooperative
Maple Valley
Meadow Ridge Farm
Miller's Biodiversity Farm
Miller's Organic Farm
Roth Sugar Bush
Russell organic
Selina Naturally
Shady Maple Farms organic
Shiloh Farms
Stannard Farm
Tropical Traditions
Whole Foods organic
Willow Run Dairy

9. Beverages

Make Your Own   Fresh   Bring Your Own

So, what will quench your thirst? As with every other item on your grocery list, you have a variety of choices when it comes to what you drink. For those who have access to safe drinking water, tap water will always remain the best choice. It is sugar-free, calorie-free, and easy on the budget. Add a little fresh fruit to the glass to enhance the flavor and make it a little more exciting!

In addition to water, every drink option should be evaluated for what has been added to it, such as additives, colors, sugar, artificial sweeteners, or preservatives. As with other items on your grocery list, try to make your own drinks to ensure that you are getting the purest product and avoiding the artificial ingredients.

Sugar - Consuming high-sugar drinks leads to weight gain, increased risk of developing type 2 diabetes, heart disease, and gout.[108]

Beware of sugar. One 12 oz. soda contains an average of 8 teaspoons of sugar![109] That is more than the daily recommended amount in just one drink! According to the American Heart Association, women should have less than 6 teaspoons of sugar and sweeteners per day, while men should have less than 9 teaspoons.[110]

High-Fructose Corn Syrup - Every aisle in the grocery store, including beverages, has products filled with high-fructose corn syrup because it's cheaper than using sugar. It increases the risk for diabetes and blocks our body's signal to the brain indicating that we are full; as a result, we overeat (and we wonder why the obesity rate is so high).[111]

Artificial Sweeteners/Additives - Avoid ingredients such as sodium benzoate, urethane, sulfur dioxide, and aspartame, just to name a few, as these are linked to cancer, asthma, rashes, hyperactivity, and fainting.[112] Food and drink preservatives are, unfortunately, unavoidable for grocery store foods. Without them foods would rot and mold before they even reached the shelves. At the risk of sounding too dramatic, the consequences of these chemicals can be deadly, as research is continuing to investigate the links with cancer, seizures, obesity, and migraines.[113]

Coffee

What Should I Look For?
- Highly quality beans
- Brands using shade-grown methods

What Should I Limit?
- Pesticides

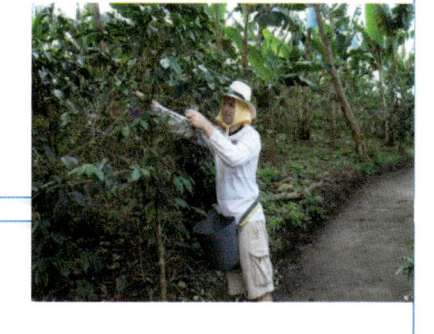

Juice

What Should I Look For?
- Make your own
- Organic
- 100% juice
- Carbonated juices made without added sugar

What Should I Limit?
- Artificial Sweeteners: Equal, NutraSweet, or Splenda
- Additives, dyes, or preservatives
- 100% natural

The Weston A. Price Foundation recommends the following brands. For more brands and suggestions, go to www.westonaprice.org[114]

Example Brands to Buy
Cultures for Health cultured vegetable juices
Earth in Common Grainfields B.E. fermented drinks (wholegrain, lemon, and ginger)
Kanne bread drink
Wise Choice Market cultured vegetable juices
Zukay vegetable kvasses

Kombucha

What Should I Look For?
🛒 Organic
🛒 Made with organic black tea

⚠ What Should I Limit?
🛒 Artificial flavors or non-organic

The Weston A. Price Foundation recommends the following brands. For more brands and suggestions, go to www.westonaprice.org.

Example Brands to Buy
Aqua Vitea
Copper Creek Farms
GT's organic raw
Meadow Ridge Farm
Miller's Organic Farm
ProNatura
Rocky Plains, LLP
The Rejuvenation Co.
Willow Run Dairy

74

Soda

What Should I Look For?
🛒 Organic

⚠️ What Should I Limit?
🛒 High-fructose corn syrup
🛒 Artificial sweeteners: NutraSweet, Equal, Splenda, aspartame, or sucralose

The Weston A. Price Foundation recommends the following brands. For more brands and suggestions, go to www.westonaprice.org.[115]

Example Brands to Buy
Burgie's Organics kefir soda   **Willow Run ginger ale**
Miller's Organic Farm ginger ale

Sport Drinks

What Should I Look For?
🛒 Make your own
🛒 Organic

⚠️ What Should I Limit?
🛒 Non-organic
🛒 Added sweeteners
🛒 Have in moderation (most contain more sugar than a serving of soda)

Tea and Ice Tea

What Should I Look For?
- Organic loose leaf tea
- Organic tea bags, unbleached bags
- Tea ball instead of tea bag

What Should I Limit?
- Added sweeteners or flavors
- GMO ingredients (corn starch, soy lecithin, etc.)
- Pyramid shaped plastic, nylon, or bleached tea bags
- Paper tea bags treated with Epichlorophydrin (EPC)

Example Brands to Buy
Numi
Rishi
Traditional Medicinals

Water and Bottled Water

What Should I Look For?
- Fill up your own water bottle with tap water

What Should I Limit?
- Waters with added sweeteners
- BPA plastic bottles
- Vitamin water (sugar, artificial sweeteners, flavors)

Our Recommendations

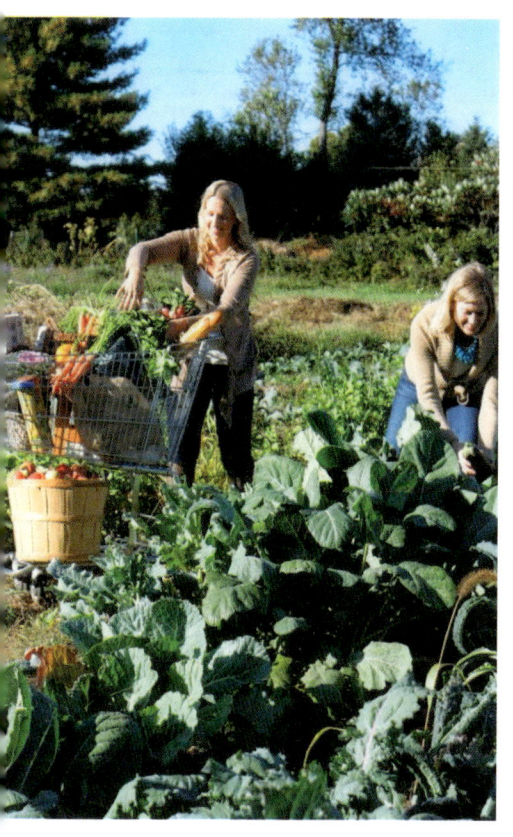

🍽 Bake and cook when time permits.

🍽 Try to buy the healthiest foods for you and your family.

🍽 Purchase at least 50% of your groceries outside the store. Join a CSA for meat, eggs, and produce.

🍽 Allow flexibility. Eat healthy 80% of the time, and allow 20% for treats, eating out, etc.

Dr. Phil Howard, an Assistant Professor at Michigan State University, created a chart to show the organic industry ownership. See the chart on the next page. This chart shows many commonly found organic brands and how they are tied to the top food producers in North America. Businesses change ownership all of the time. A food that was once produced by a small, family-owned company who valued high-quality, organic practices can be bought out by a larger company that might change to more cost-efficient ingredients to increase shelf life and speed up production rates. Just as it is important for you to know your farmer, it is important that you know who is making your food, and the values that are set by those companies.
To see more charts, go to
https://www.msu.edu/~howardp/organicindustry.html.

Organic Industry Structure:
Acquisitions & Alliances, Top 100 Food Processors in North America

Snyder's-Lance #61
- Late July (December 2007 minority stake)

Perdue Farms #27
- Coleman Natural (May 2011)
  - Hans (August 2003)
  - Petaluma/Rosie (January 2002)
- Draper Valley Farms (August 2007)

Hershey Foods #20
- Dagoba (October 2006)

Campbell Soup Co. #30
- Plum Organics (May 2013)
- Bolthouse Farms (July 2012, $1.55 B)
  - Wolfgang Puck (July 2008)

M&M Mars #10
- Bloomfield Bakers
- Seeds of Change (1997)

Mondelez (spinoff from #4 Kraft in 2012)
- Boca Foods (February 2000)
- Back to Nature (September 2003 100% Equity; August 2012 majority stake sold to Brynwood Partners)
- Green & Black's (January 2010)

Hain Celestial #82
- Frutti di Bosco / Millina's Finest (June 2001)
- Walnut Acres (October 2001)
- Mountain Sun / ShariAnn's (June 2003)
- MaraNatha / SunSpire
- Ella's Kitchen (May 2013)
- BluePrint (November 2012)
- TofuTown (June 2007 From Dean)
- Westbrae / Bearitos / Westsoy / Little Bear (October 1997, $23.5 M)
- Celestial Seasonings (March 2000, $390 M)

JAB/D.E. Master Blenders (formerly #28 Sara Lee)
- Tea Forte (January 2012)
- Peet's Coffee & Tea (August 2012, $1 B)

Dean #7
- White Wave/Silk (May 2002 $189 M; May 2013 Spinoff, 0% Equity)
- Alta Dena (May 1999)
- Horizon (July 1998 13% Equity; January 2004 100% Equity $216 M)
- The Organic Cow of Vermont (April 1999)

Hillshire Brands (formerly #28 Sara Lee)
- Aidell's Sausage (May 2011, $87 M)

Nestle #3
- Sweet Leaf Tea (May 2011)
- Tribe Mediterranean Foods (September 2008 $57M via Israeli subsidiary Osem Group (50.1% Equity))

Coca-Cola #11
- Honest Tea (February 2008 40% Equity $43 M; March 2011 100% Equity)
- Odwalla (October 2001, $181 M)

Pepsi #1
- Naked Juice (November 2006)

Miller-Coors #17
- Crispin (February 2012)
- Fox Barrel (January 2010)

Diamond Foods #88
- Kettle (February 2010 $615 M)

Maple Leaf Foods #24 — 90% Equity

Canada Bread Co. #63
- Olafson Baking (July 2002)

Phil Howard, Associate Professor
Michigan State University

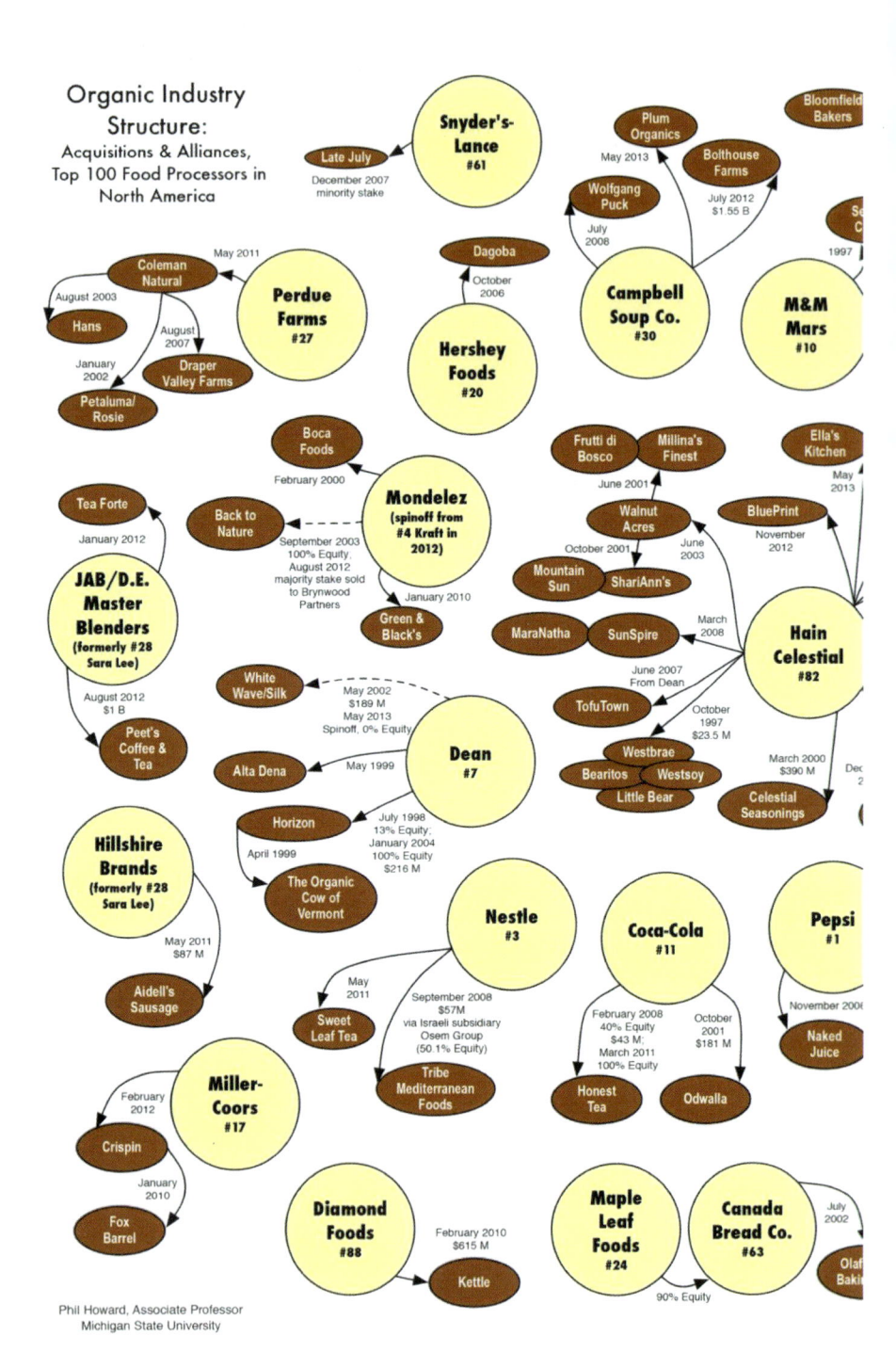

78

May 2013

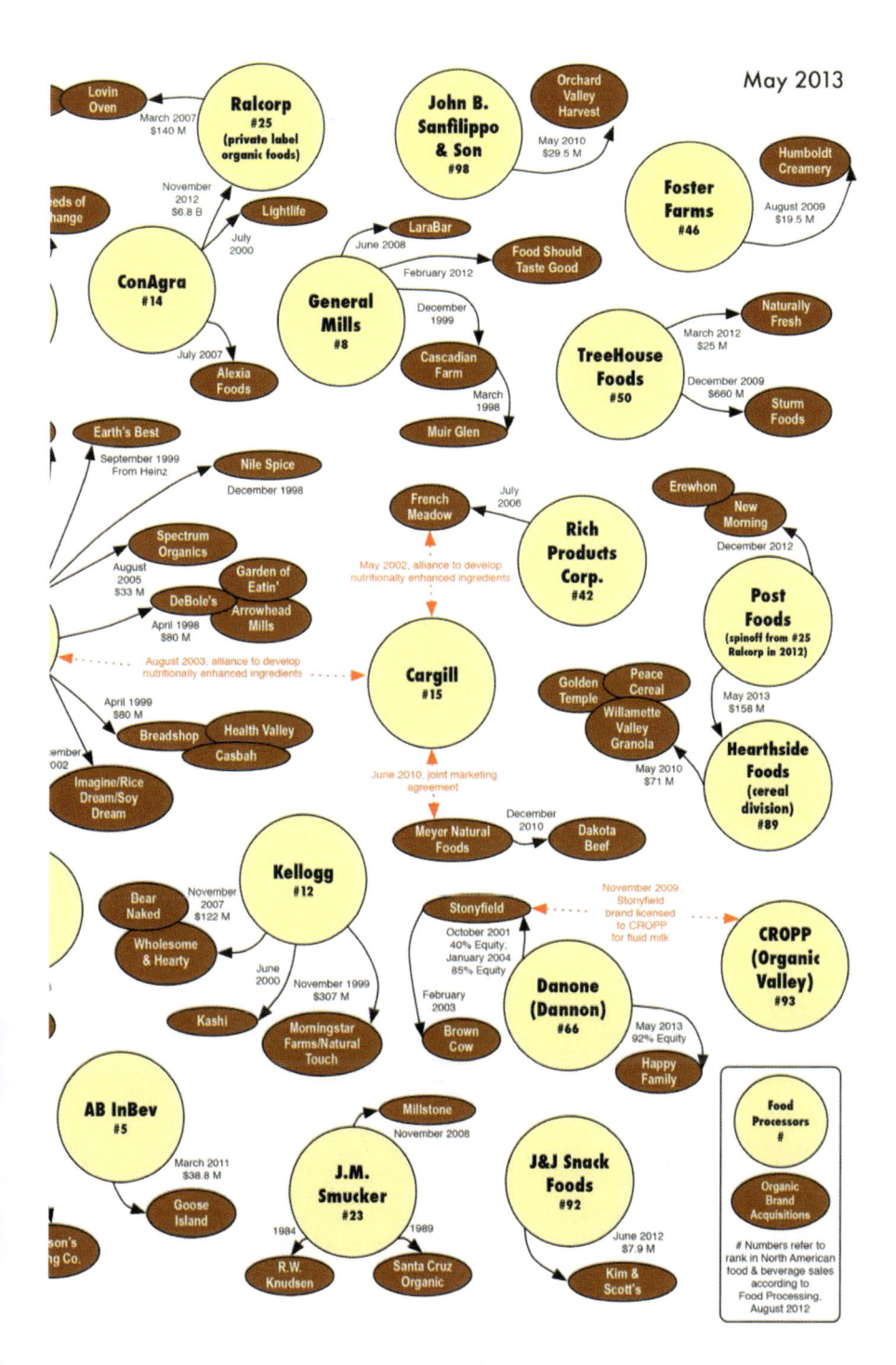

Food Processor Organic Brand Acquisitions Map

ConAgra #14
- Lovin' Oven — March 2007, $140 M
- Ralcorp #25 (private label organic foods) — November 2012, $6.8 B
- Lightlife — July 2000
- Alexia Foods — July 2007
- Seeds of Change

Ralcorp #25 (private label organic foods)

John B. Sanfilippo & Son #98
- Orchard Valley Harvest — May 2010, $29.5 M

Foster Farms #46
- Humboldt Creamery — August 2009, $19.5 M

General Mills #8
- LaraBar — June 2008
- Food Should Taste Good — February 2012
- Cascadian Farm — December 1999
- Muir Glen — March 1998

TreeHouse Foods #50
- Naturally Fresh — March 2012, $25 M
- Sturm Foods — December 2009, $660 M

Heinz
- Earth's Best — September 1999, From Heinz
- Nile Spice — December 1998
- Spectrum Organics — August 2005, $33 M
- Garden of Eatin'
- DeBole's — April 1998, $80 M
- Arrowhead Mills
- Breadshop — April 1999, $80 M
- Health Valley
- Casbah
- Imagine/Rice Dream/Soy Dream

August 2003, alliance to develop nutritionally enhanced ingredients

Rich Products Corp. #42
- French Meadow — July 2006

May 2002, alliance to develop nutritionally enhanced ingredients

Cargill #15

June 2010, joint marketing agreement

- Meyer Natural Foods
- Dakota Beef — December 2010

Post Foods (spinoff from #25 Ralcorp in 2012)
- Erewhon
- New Morning — December 2012
- Golden Temple
- Peace Cereal
- Willamette Valley Granola
- Hearthside Foods (cereal division) #89 — May 2013, $158 M — May 2010, $71 M

Kellogg #12
- Bear Naked — November 2007, $122 M
- Wholesome & Hearty
- Kashi — June 2000
- Morningstar Farms/Natural Touch — November 1999, $307 M
- Stonyfield — October 2001 40% Equity; January 2004 85% Equity
- Brown Cow — February 2003

Danone (Dannon) #66
- Happy Family — May 2013, 92% Equity

November 2009, Stonyfield brand licensed to CROPP for fluid milk

CROPP (Organic Valley) #93

AB InBev #5
- Goose Island — March 2011, $38.8 M
- Anheuser-Busch Co.

J.M. Smucker #23
- Millstone — November 2008
- R.W. Knudsen — 1984
- Santa Cruz Organic — 1989

J&J Snack Foods #92
- Kim & Scott's — June 2012, $7.9 M

Legend:
- Food Processors #
- Organic Brand Acquisitions
- # Numbers refer to rank in North American food & beverage sales according to Food Processing, August 2012

79

Recommended Reading

Animal, Vegetable, Miracle, Barbara Kingsolver, Camille Kingsolver, and Steven L. Hopp
CAFO: The Tragedy of Industrial Animal Factories, Daniel Imhoff
Eating Animals, Jonathan Safran Foer
Folks, This Ain't Normal, Joel Salatin
Harmony, The Prince of Wales
Harvest, Nicola Smith
In Defense of Food, Michael Pollan
Jamie's Food Revolution, Jamie Oliver
Make the Bread, Buy the Butter, Jennifer Reese
Nutrition and Physical Degeneration, Weston Andrew Price
Sunfood Living, John McCabe
The End of Overeating, Kessler, David
The Omnivore's Dilemma, Michael Pollan
The World According to Monsanto, Marie-Monique Robin

Movies

Black Gold
Food, Inc.
Fresh
Future of Food

Genetic Roulette
Hungry for Change
Peaceful Kingdom
Queen of the Sun

Tapped
The Real Life of Farmer John

Apps

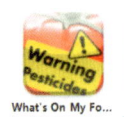

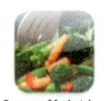

What's On My Fo... (Pesticide Action Net...)
Seafood Watch (Monterey Bay Aquari...)
Farmers Market L... (Whagaa Software Inc.)
Dirty Dozen (Environmental Work...)
True Food (True Food Network)

Glossary

Additives: Man-made laboratory chemicals added to foods to enhance the color, flavor, and texture of foods, as well as to prolong shelf life.

Antibiotic Resistance: The ability of a bacteria or virus to withstand the effects of an antibiotic. If a person develops a resistance, the antibiotics will no longer work to kill the bug and cure symptoms.

Antibiotics: Medications given to animals to fight off bacterial illnesses and prolong their life until they make it to your table. Some factory farms routinely give antibiotics as a preventative for disease in animals.

Artificial Flavors: Man-made laboratory chemicals added to foods to enhance or imitate their flavors. They help to mimic the taste of sweet, sour, tart, smoky, spicy, etc.

Aspartame: An artificial, man-made sweetener. It is a low-calorie, non-sugar sweetener and is also known as Equal® and NutraSweet®.

Bisphenol A (BPA): A chemical used in certain types of plastics, lining of metal cans, bottle tops, and many other products. BPA mimics estrogen in the body and affects the endocrine system. Studies have shown that exposure to BPA increases ill health effects of the brain, behavior, and prostate of fetuses, infants, and children.

Cane Sugar: A sweet substance that has been extracted from the sugar plant (sugarcane). It can be processed into a variety of sugars and sugar substitutes; raw sugar, however, tends to be the most expensive with the most amount of flavor.

Community Supported Agriculture (CSA): A way for consumers to buy beef, poultry, eggs, and seasonal fruits and vegetables directly from a local farmer instead of from the grocery store. The farmer delivers the order weekly, or monthly, to a neighborhood host location. Farmers benefit because they receive payment early in the season to help with their cash flow, and they also "cultivate" a relationship with the people who eat their food. Consumers benefit by getting to know the farmer who grows their food, while buying food at its freshest, full of flavor and vitamins. Consumers are exposed to new vegetables and a new way of cooking and are able to learn how their food is grown. CSA's are usually family-run farms and they invite their members out to the farm at least once a season. This is a great way to buy directly from the farmer.

Concentrated Animal Feeding Operations (CAFO's): A farm that operates as a business raising a large number of animals in a small space for the purpose of selling the animal for food. These farms operate with profit as their primary goal and often disregard sanitary conditions, resulting in the spread of disease among the animals. The animals are often mistreated and live in a confined area with feed, manure, urine, and dead animals. The animals eat the feed that consists of ground GMO corn, soy, and other waste materials, mixed with antibiotics. The sick animals are given antibiotics to gain weight and slow infection so they can reach slaughterhouse weight quickly. Some are given hormones to ensure that the animals grow faster and that more milk is produced in a shorter amount of time. CAFO's are also called factory farms.

Conventional Farming: Farming that uses pesticides, GMO's, feed additives, antibiotics and growth hormones.

Cornucopia Institute: A non-profit organization based in Wisconsin. They support family farmers and provide education to the public through research and investigation of food issues.

Crop Rotation: The pattern of growing different crops each season in the same field of land. This rotation helps boost soil structure and fertility by replenishing the soil's nutrients, such as nitrogen; keeps the soil healthy; and helps to decrease the amount of pests and pathogens that appear when the same crop is grown year after year. This practice helps provide more minerals and vitamins to the produce you consume, compared to the farmers who do not use crop rotation.

Environmental Working Group (EWG): A non-profit organization that develops guides and resources based on their research. They have a website that provides information about what is happening with beauty products, food, and the environment.

Epichlorohydrin (ECH): a liquid, moderately soluble in water, used to make plastics and glues. When ECH comes in contact with water, it changes to a different compound. It is found in tea bag and sausage casings. It can lead to cancer and fertility problems in males.

Factory Farms: see Concentrated Animal Feeding Operations.

Family Farm: A farm owned and operated by a family to produce food, grain, or livestock. These farms are managed for the well-being of the people as well as animals, and not solely for profit. These animals and foods are raised on the pasture without growth hormones and only receive antibiotics when ill. They raise a wide range of animal breeds. Ask the farmer about his farming practices to know you are getting the healthiest products.

Farmers Market: A place where local farmers come together to sell their fresh fruits, vegetables, eggs, cheese, home-made breads, flowers, and plants to consumers. The link card is accepted at farmers markets.

Fermented Foods: Fermentation is an effective means of food preservation. There are many health benefits from fermented foods. It helps destroy toxins so that all of the healthy vitamins, minerals, and beneficial bacteria are better absorbed by the body. Some common fermented foods are pickles, sauerkraut, vinegar, yogurt, cheese, coffee, chocolate, sausage, and salami.

Fillers: Substances added to foods to make a heavier product, so it can be sold at a cheaper price. Basically, you are not eating a product with 100 percent of the raw material.

Food Co-op: A food-buying club created by individuals who purchase groceries from food distributors. Together, the club chooses these food suppliers (farmers, companies) based on their values and farming practices so that they are purchasing the highest quality of food. Members receive discounts on the foods they purchase.

Genetically Modified Organisms (GMO's): An animal, fish or seed that has been purposefully, scientifically modified for a desirable trait, a trait that would not have occurred naturally in nature. This is different than hybridization. Crops are altered in such ways to resist pests, insects, herbicides, and harsh environmental conditions by designing a seed with pesticide resistant properties. Due to the abundance of GMO corn and GMO soy in many processed foods, GMO's are found in ***almost every*** product! These GMO foods are not labeled as "GMO" in the United States. Some examples of GMO foods are soy, cottonseed, corn, canola, U.S. Papaya, alfalfa, and sugar. Many countries in the European Union, as well as Saudi Arabia, Algeria, and Brazil, just to name a few ban GMO foods and label foods that contain GMO's.

Green Polka Dot Box: An online grocery store that sells natural, organic, and non-GMO foods at great prices. The green box with polka dots is delivered to your home.

Growth Hormones (rBGH): A man-made (genetically engineered) substitute for a growth hormone that is naturally produced by cows. It is also called Posilac. Farmers inject their cows with it to increase milk production. When we consume milk or dairy products with rBGH, we are consuming these extra hormones.

Herbicide: A chemical used to kill plants and weeds.

Hexane: A bi-product of gasoline used as a solvent to separate the soybean and proteins. It is considered a toxic to the nerves.

High-fructose corn syrup: Natural corn syrup that is changed in a laboratory to make it sweeter. It is less expensive than sugar, so it is used in many processed foods and sodas. It is commonly used in breads, lunch meats, yogurts, and cereals.

Insecticide: A chemical substance used to kill insects.

Irradiation: The application of ionizing radiation to food to improve the shelf life and to kill organisms or insects that may be on the food.

Lean Finely Textured Beef (LFTB): Also called pink slime, has been added to ground beef since 2001. This product is made from connective tissue and fat, and is treated with ammonium to kill bacteria. Products that contain LFTB are not labeled. This is found in meat sold at supermarkets and restaurants.

Marine Stewardship Council (MSC): MSC is the world's leading ecolabel and certification program for wild-caught seafood. When consumers see the blue MSC ecolabel they can be sure that product is traceable back to a fishery that has been certified to the MSC's rigorous environmental standard as a sustainable and well-managed fishery. The standard ensures the fish stocks are healthy, the impact of fishing on the marine ecosystem is minimal, and the fishery is well-managed.

Mercury: A chemical element that occurs in the environment, but is released into the air through industrial pollution. It turns into methyl mercury while in the water and is then absorbed by algae on the low end of the food chain. Fish absorb the methyl mercury as they feed in these waters. It is this type of mercury that can be harmful to our health.

Monosodium Glutamate (MSG): Used in processed foods to enhance flavor. It is found in foods that have a long shelf life.

Monterey Bay Aquarium: the Monterey Bay Aquarium Seafood Watch program creates science-based recommendations that help consumers and businesses make ocean-friendly seafood choices.

Natural: A term that does not have a regulated definition like organic. It may contain pesticides, GMO's, antibiotics, hormones, and irradiation.

Nitrates: A substance used to preserve meats and processed foods to prevent bacteria from growing. It may be linked to cancer.

Non-GMO Project: a non-profit organization dedicated to educate consumers about non-GMO foods and give them verified non-GMO options at the grocery store. The organization is dedicated to saving the non-GMO food supply and believe everyone should have an informed choice about whether or not to consume GMO's.

Non-Organic: Grown or made <u>with</u> pesticides, GMO seeds, irradiation, antibiotics, food additives, growth hormones, or artificial chemicals.

Organic: Grown or made <u>without</u> pesticides, GMO seeds, irradiation, antibiotics, food additives, growth hormones, or artificial chemicals.

PAN (Pesticide Action Network): An organization that finds sustainable methods to use in farming instead of pesticides.

Partially Hydrogenated Oils: Another word for trans-fat.

Pasteurization: The process by which milk is heated to a high temperature to destroy certain germs and to help prevent the milk from souring during its shelf life. The high heat also kills good germs and nutrients, like lactic acid bacilli (your body's good yeast) and vitamin C. Research supports the belief that milk does not have to be pasteurized and that a person will not become ill from raw milk.

Pesticides: A chemical sprayed on food crops or animals to deter any unwanted pests. Fruits and vegetables sprayed with pesticides are called non-organic. Some studies have linked the use of pesticides to cancer, skin conditions, and organ damage, since the pesticide cannot be fully washed off.

Polychlorinated Biphenyl (PCB's): A chemical used in a variety of things, such as coolant fluid, until it was banned in the United States in 1979. PCB's are still found in our environment and in fish. They are linked to cancer and other health problems.

Preservative: A chemical added to a food to prevent decay.

rBST (rBGH): recombinant bovine somatotropin, a man-made growth hormone that is used in some dairy cows. rBST is a hormone that naturally is produced in a cow's pituitary gland for metabolic process regulation. Major companies created a synthetic version of the hormone in the lab, which is injected into the cow so they produce more milk. It is banned in Canada, Australia, Japan, Israel, New Zealand, and the European Union.

Saturated Fat: A fat that contains only saturated fatty acids, is solid at room temperature, and comes primarily from animal food products. Some examples of saturated fat are butter, lard, meat fat, solid shortening, palm oil, and coconut oil.

Sodium Nitrite: Maintains the red color in meat. For example, hot dogs would look gray without it.

Trans Fat: (*trans* fatty acids, industrial trans fats, or partially hydrogenated oils): A fatty acid produced by the partial hydrogenation of vegetable oils and present in hardened vegetable oils, most margarines, commercial baked foods, and many fried foods. An excess of these fats in the diet is linked to increase in cholesterol levels.

Ultra-pasteurization: The process by which milk is heated to an even higher temperature than pasteurized milk, which extends the shelf life to six to nine months. This changes the taste and textures, so thickening agents are added to bring back the original viscosity. Many of the vitamins and minerals are destroyed in this process.

Unfermented Soy: Soy that has not been fermented, such as modern day soy products, GMO soy, and all those soy ingredients added to foods. Some believe it is linked to digestive irritability, a compromised immune system, PMS, endometriosis, infertility, allergies, and ADHD.

USDA Organic Sticker: products with this sticker contain at least 95–99% organic ingredients.

Weston A. Price Foundation: nonprofit organization founded by Sally Fallon and Mary G. Eniga, based on the teachings of Dr. Weston A. Price, a dentist who believed that health stems from eating traditional sources of foods with the most nutrients.

Index

Baby foods 48-50
Baking powder 48-51
Beef 18-20
Bottle water 72-73, 76
Bread 48-50, 51
Butter 33-35
Cake mix 48-50, 52
Candy 48-50, 52-53
Cereal 48-50, 53-54
Cheese 33-36
Chicken (poultry) 21-24
Chips 48-50, 55
Chocolate 48-50, 52-53
Coconut 48-50, 56
Coffee 72-73
Cookies 48-50, 57
Cottage cheese 33-34, 37
Crackers 48-50, 58
Cream cheese 33-34, 37
Dairy 33-42
Eggs 43-47
Fish 25-28
Flour 48-50, 59
Frozen dinner 48-50, 59
Fruit 14-17
Granola bars 48-50, 59-60
Honey 48-50, 61
Ice tea 72-73, 76
Ice cream 33-34, 38-39
Jam 48-50, 61

Juice 72-74
Kombucha 72-73, 74
Margarine 33-35
Meat (beef) 18-20
Milk 33-34, 40-41
Miso 29-32
Muffins 48-50, 62
Nut butter 48-50, 64
Nutrition bars 48-50, 59-60
Oils 48-50, 62-63
Pancake mix 48-50, 63
Pasta 48-50, 63
Pasta sauce 48-50, 64
Peanut butter 48-50, 64
Popcorn 48-50, 65
Seeds 48-50, 65
Soda 72-73, 75
Soups 48-50, 66
Soy products 29-32
Sport drinks 72-73, 75
Sugar 48-50, 66-71
Sweeteners 48-50, 66-71
Syrup 48-50, 71
Tea 72-73, 76
Tempeh 29-32
Tofu 29-32
Vegetables 14-17
Water 72-73, 76
Yogurt 33-34, 42

References

"2002 Census of Agriculture." *U.S. Department of Agriculture*, June 2004; retrieved February 23, 2012, http://www. usda.gov

"Additives." *Sustainable Table Food Program*, 2013; retrieved October 3, 2013, http://www.sustainabletable.org/385/additives

"Adult Obesity Facts." *Centers for Disease Control and Prevention*, August 16, 2013; retrieved August 20, 2013, http://www.cdc.gov/obesity/data/adult.html

"Bald chicken 'needs no plucking." *BBC News*, May 21, 2012; retrieved April 4, 2013, http://news.bbc.co.uk/2/hi/sci/tech/2000003.stm

"Boys--like girls--hitting puberty earlier." *CCN Health*, October 23, 2012; retrieved September 20, 2013, http://www.cnn.com/2012/10/20/health/boys-early-puberty/index.html

"Chickens Used for Food." *People for the Ethical Treatment of Animals*, retrieved June 10, 2013, http://www.peta.org/issues/animals-used-for-food/chickens.aspx

"Dairy Production on Factory Farms." *Farm Sanctuary*, retrieved September 24, 2013, http://www.farmsanctuary.org/learn/factory-farming/dairy

Daley, C., Abbott, A., Doyle, P., Nader, G., & Larson, S. (2010). A review of fatty acid profiles and antioxidant content in grass-fed and grain-fed beef. Nutrition Journal, 9:10, 1-12.

"Diabetes Facts and Figures." *Diabetes Prevention and Control Coalition, 2012;* retrieved September 20, 2013, http://notme.com/dpca/diabetesFacts.html

"Dr. Weil's Anti-inflammatory Food Pyramid." *Dr. Weil*, 2013; retrieved October 5, 2013, http://www.drweil.com/drw/u/PAG00361/anti-inflammatory-food-pyramid.html

Du Bois, Christine M., Tan, Chee-Beng, Mintz, Sidney. *The World of Soy*. Illinois: University of Illinois, 2008.

"Egg Production on Factory Farms." *Farm Sanctuary*, retrieved July 1, 2013, http://www.farmsanctuary.org/learn/factory-farming/chickens-used-for-eggs

"European Union Bans Battery Cages for Egg-Laying Hens." *Food Safety News,* January 12, 2012; Retrieved July 2, 201, http://www.foodsafetynews.com/2012/01/european-union-bans-battery-cages-for-egg-laying-hens/#.Uk4lXBD9VdF

"EWG's 2013 Shopper's Guide to Pesticides in Produce™" *Environmental Working Group,* 2013; retrieved June 10, 2013, http://www.ewg.org/foodnews/summary.php

"Factory Farming: Cruelty to Animals." *People for the Ethical Treatment of Animals,* 2013; retrieved June 10, 2013, http://www.peta.org/issues/animals-used-for-food/factory-farming.aspx

"Fair Trade & Shade Grown Organic Coffee--A Growing Movement." *Organic Consumers Association*, retrieved September 10, 2013, http://www.organicconsumers.org/Organic/faircoffee.cfm
Foer, Jonathan Safran. *Eating Animals.* New York: Hachette Book Group, 2009

"Fishy Farms: The Government's Push for Factory Farms in Our Oceans." *Food & Water Watch,* October 12, 2011; retrieved October 1, 2013, http://www.foodandwaterwatch.org/reports/fishy-farms

"Free Range vs. Pastured: Chicken and Eggs." *Mother Earth News*, March 5, 2009; retrieved April 12, 2013, http://www.motherearthnews.com/homesteading-and-livestock/free-range-versus-pastured-chicken-and-eggs.aspx#axzz2hiuiTWej

"GE Fish." *Center for Food Safety,* June 20, 2013; retrieved May 29, 2013, http://www.centerforfoodsafety.org/issues/309/#

"Genetically Modified Foods." *American Academy of Environmental Medicine*, May 8, 2009; retrieved June 10, 2013, http://www.aaemonline.org/gmopost.html
"Getting Wild Nutrition from Modern Food." *Eat Wild,* 2008; retrieved August 12, 2011, http://www.eatwild.com/animals.html

"GMO Food, Antibiotic Laced Meat and High Fructose Corn Syrup Have Made the U.S. the Fattest Nation in History!" *Organic Consumers Association*, September 5, 2012; retrieved October 15, 2012, http://www.organicconsumers.org/articles/article_26209.cfm
Hauter, Wenonah. Foodopoly: The Battle over the Future of Food and Farming in America. New York: The New Press, 2012.

"Health Benefits of Grass-Fed Products. *"Eat Wild*, 2013; retrieved May 14, 2013, http://www.eatwild.com/healthbenefits.htm

"Health and Wellness the Trillion Dollar Industry in 2017: Key Research Highlights." *Euromonitor International,* November 29, 2012; retrieved October 3, 2013, http://blog.euromonitor.com/2012/11/health-and-wellness-the-trillion-dollar-industry-in-2017-key-research-highlights.html

"High-Fructose Corn Syrup: Not So Sweet for the Planet." *Washington Post*, March 9, 2008; retrieved September 10, 2013, http://articles.washingtonpost.com/2008-03-09/news/36881215_1_high-fructose-corn-syrup-corn-belt-hfcs

"History of Soybeans and Soy foods Worldwide: Past, Present and Future" *Soy Info Center*, 2007; retrieved August 2, 2013, http://www.soyinfocenter.com/chronologies_of_soyfoods-soymilk.php

Holtcamp, W. (2012). Obesogens. An Environmental Link to Obesity. Environmental Health Perspectives, 120:2, 63-68.

"How Sweet Is It" *Harvard School of Public Health*, 2013; retrieved September 19, 2013, http://www.hsph.harvard.edu/nutritionsource/how-sweet-is-it

"Human Health Criteria- Methylmercury Fish Tissue Criterion." *Environmental Protection Agency,* January 2001; retrieved June 1, 2013, http://water.epa.gov/scitech/swguidance/standards/criteria/aqlife/methylmercury/factsheet.cfm

"Industrial Agriculture." *Pesticide Action Network*, retrieved March 24, 2013, http://www.panna.org/issues/food-agriculture/industrial-agriculture

"Is Agribusiness Making Food Less Nutritious?" *Mother Earth News*, June/July 2004; retrieved July 2013, http://www.motherearthnews.com/real-food/is-agribusiness-making-food-less-nutritious.aspx#axzz2giRjjchb

"Labeling Organic Products." *U.S. Department of Agriculture,* October 2012; retrieved May 4, 2013, http://www.ams.usda.gov/AMSv1.0/getfile?dDocName=STELDEV3004446&acct=nopgeninfo

"Labels that tell you a little." *Food & Water Watch*, 2007; retrieved April 29, 2013, http://www.foodandwaterwatch.org/food/consumer-labels/labels-that-tell-you-a-little

"Local Harvest" *Local Harvest,* 2012; retrieved August 13, 20012, http://www.localharvest.org

Love, D.C, Halden, R.U., Davis, M.F. and Nachman, K.E. "Feather Meal: A Previously Unrecognized Route for Reentry into the Food Supply of Multiple Pharmaceuticals and Personal Care Products (PPCPS)." *Environmental Science & Technology*, Vol. 46, 3795-3802, March 21, 2012, http://pubs.acs.org/doi/pdf/10.1021/es203970e

"Mandatory Labeling for GE Salmon Overcomes Major Hurdle." retrieved June 29, 2013, http://www.non-gmoreport.com/articles/sept10/non-GMO_food_soybean_seed_breeding_programs.php

McCabe, John and Wolfe, David. *Sunfood Living: Resource Guide for Global Health.* California: Sunfood Publishing, 2007.
"Meet Real Free-Range Eggs." *Mother Earth News*, October/November 2007; retrieved May 29, 2013, http://www.motherearthnews.com/homesteading-and-livestock/eggs-zl0z0703zswa.aspx#axzz2ghFZpmv3

"Menstruation and the Menstrual Cycle Fact Sheet." *Office on Women's Health, U.S. Health and Human Services*, October 21, 2009; retrieved September 10, 2013, http://womenshealth.gov/publications/our-publications/fact-sheet/menstruation.cfm

"Mental Disorders Skyrocket: Try This To Avoid Becoming The Next Victim" *Mercola.com,* June 20, 2013; retrieved August 5, 2013, http://articles.mercola.com/sites/articles/archive/2013/06/20/children-mental-disorder.aspx

"Natural and Organic Foods." *FDA, Food Marketing Institute,* retrieved July 1, 2013, http://www.fda.gov/ohrms/dockets/dockets/06p0094/06p-0094-cp00001-05-Tab-04-Food-Marketing-Institute-vol1.pdf
"Natural beef can come from cows given added hormones or antibiotics." *The Cornucopia Institute,* September 30, 2013; retrieved October 1, 2013, http://www.cornucopia.org/2013/09/natural-meat-labels-confuse-shoppers

"Overweight and Obesity Data and Statistics." *Centers for Disease Control and Prevention,* January 11, 2013; retrieved February 12, 2013, http://www.cdc.gov/obesity/data/childhood.html

"Pan Pesticides Database – Pesticide Products." *Pesticide Action Network,* 2010; retrieved September 20, 2012, http://www.pesticideinfo.org

"Pesticide News Story: EPA releases report containing latest estimates of pesticide use in the United States." *United States Environmental Protection Agency,* 2011; retrieved September 20, 2012, http://www.epa.gov/oppfead1/cb/csb_page/updates/2011/sales-usage06-07.html

Pollan, Michael. *Food Rule: Eater's Manual.* New York: Penguin Group, 2009.

"Public Health." *Public Health, 2013;* retrieved September 20, 2013 http://www.sustainabletable.org/270/public-health.

Price, Weston A., MS., D.D.S., F.A.G.D. *Nutrition and Physical Degeneration, 8th edition.* Price Pottenger Nutrition, 2008.

Price, Weston A. Foundation. *Shopping Guide 2013.* Washington, DC: Weston A. Price Foundation, 2013.

"Rainforest Alliance Certified Coffee." *Rainforest Alliance,* 2013, retrieved August 3, 2010, http://www.rainforest-alliance.org/agriculture/crops/coffee

"rBGH: What the Research Shows" *Food and Water Watch*, 2007; retrieved April 29, 2013, http://www.foodandwaterwatch.org/factsheet/what-research-shows

"Recombinant Bovine Growth Hormone." *American Cancer Society*, February 18, 2011; retrieved March 21, 2011, http://www.cancer.org/cancer/cancercauses/othercarcinogens/athome/recombinant-bovine-growth-hormone

"Russia Bans U.S. Poultry Over Chlorine." *Food Safety News*, January 7, 2010; retrieved May 16, 2013, http://www.foodsafetynews.com/2010/01/russia-bans-us-poultry-over-chlorine/#.Uk3jMBD9VdF

Robbins, John. The Food Revolution: How Your Diet Can Help Save Your Life and Our World. San Francisco: Red Wheel/Weiser, 2011.

Robin, Marie-Monique. *The World According to Monsanto: Pollution, Corruption, and the Control of the World's Food Supply.* New York: The New Press, 2010.

Salatin, Joel. *Folks, This Aint Normal A Farmer's Advice for Happier Hens, Healthier People, and A Better World. New York: Hachette Book Group, 2011.*

"Select a Seafood Watch Pocket Guide." *Monterey Bay Aquarium Seafood Watch*, Fall/Winter 2013; retrieved October 1, 2013, http://www.montereybayaquarium.org/cr/cr_seafoodwatch/download

"Soybeans." *George Mateljan Foundation,* retrieved October 10, 2013, http://www.whfoods.com/genpage.php?tname=foodspice&dbid=79

"Sugars and Carbohydrates." *American Heart Association,* September 11, 2013; retrieved September 19, 2013, http://www.heart.org/HEARTORG/GettingHealthy/NutritionCenter/HealthyDietGoals/Sugars-and-Carbohydrates_UCM_303296_Article.jsp

"Sugary Drinks and Obesity Fact Sheet." *Harvard School of Public Health*, 2013; retrieved September 19, 2013, http://www.hsph.harvard.edu/nutritionsource/sugary-drinks-fact-sheet

"Survey finds many non-GMO food soybean seed breeding programs." *The Organic and Non-GMO Report,* September 2010;

"The Basics: Antibiotic Resistance." *Keep Antibiotics Working,* December 4, 2003; retrieved May 29, 2013, http://www.keepantibioticsworking.com/new/basics.php

"The Basics: Antibiotic Resistance." *Keep Antibiotics Working,* December 4, 2003; retrieved January 10, 2011, http://www.keepantibioticsworking.com/new/basics.php

"The Cruelest of All Factory Farm Products: Eggs From Caged Hens." *The Huffington Post,* January 14, 2013; retrieved March 30, 2013, http://www.huffingtonpost.com/bruce-friedrich/eggs-from-caged-hens_b_2458525.html

"The Dangers of High Fructose Corn Syrup." *Diabetes Health,* August 20, 2008; retrieved September 30, 2013, http://diabeteshealth.com/read/2008/08/20/4274/the-dangers-of-high-fructose-corn-syrup

"The hidden salt in chicken." *L.A. Times,* June 22, 2009; retrieved June 4, 2013, http://articles.latimes.com/2009/jun/22/health/he-nutrition22

"Trans Fats: The Science and the Risks" *WebMD,* July 6, 2006; retrieved May 1, 2013, http://www.webmd.com/diet/features/trans-fats-science-and-risks

"Ultra-Pasteurized Milk." Linda Joyce Forristal, CTA, MTA, The Weston A. Price Foundation, May 23, 2004; retrieved May 29, 2011, http://www.westonaprice.org/modern-foods/ultra-pasteurized-milk

"U.S. National Cancer Institute Manipulates Cancer Statistics." *Cancer Prevention Coalition,* 2013; retrieved September 20, 2013, http://www.preventcancer.com/losing/nci/manipulates.htm

Weber, Karl and Participant Media. *Food, Inc.* New York: Public Affairs, 2009

"What Does Organic Mean?" *California Certified Organic Farmers (CCOF)*, 2013; retrieved June 29, 2013, http://www.ccof.org/ccof/media-room/fact-sheets

"What is a GMO?" *Non-GMO Project*, 2013; retrieved April 4, 2013, http://www.nongmoproject.org/learn-more/what-is-gmo

"What is High-Fructose Corn Syrup? What are the health concerns?" *Mayo Clinic, September 27, 2012;* retrieved June 3, 2013, http://www.mayoclinic.com/health/high-fructose-corn-syrup/AN01588

"What's Wrong with Food Irradiation?" *Organic Consumers Association,* retrieved March 24, 2013, http://www.organicconsumers.org/Irrad/irradfact.cfm

"Women and Heart Disease Fact Sheet." *Centers for Disease Control and Prevention, August 22, 2013;* retrieved September 20, 2013, http://www.cdc.gov/dhdsp/data_statistics/fact_sheets/fs_women_heart

About the Authors

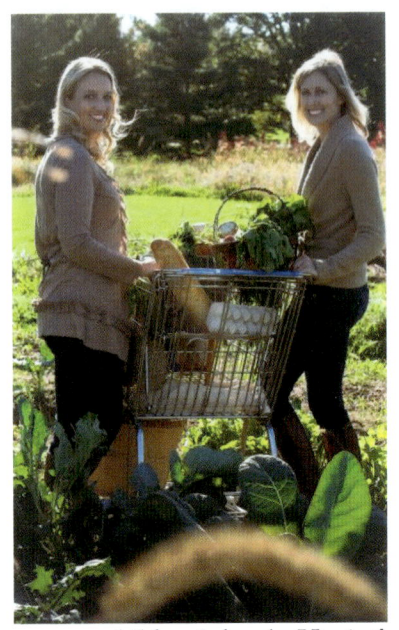

Jennifer Lucas is a pediatric nurse and Family Nurse Practitioner who believes knowing where your food comes from is the best way to promote health. Jennifer pursued her Bachelor of Science in Nursing at Loyola University in Chicago and worked as a Registered Nurse on the Pediatric Unit at Loyola Medical Center. She also worked in a wellness clinic assisting with weight loss and health promotion. After completing her Masters of Science in Nursing, she worked in primary care as a Family Nurse Practitioner. Jennifer currently teaches full-time at Loyola University Chicago in the Health Promotion Department. She wrote a children's book, *Howie the Healthy Hound*. She speaks to health care groups throughout the country on various nutrition topics. Jennifer is a Food Practitioner and President of Healthy Farm, Plate, You, LLC.

Jaclyn Taverna is a pediatric nurse and Family Nurse Practitioner who believes that food and nutrition are the basis and culprit of every disease state. Jaclyn has a Food Science and Human Nutrition degree from the University of Illinois at Urbana-Champaign. While studying to become a dietitian, she learned how to counsel a variety of patients on food choices to help them feel better. She found herself investigating the reverse. How do certain foods make us sick and how can we prevent illness from the start? To further connect these ideas, she pursued her Bachelor of Science in Nursing at Loyola University Chicago, where she worked as a Registered Nurse on the Pediatric Unit at Loyola University Medical Center. Since completing her Masters of Science in Nursing she has worked as a Family Nurse Practitioner in the primary care setting, as well as at a nutrition and weight loss clinic. Currently she works at an Allergy and Asthma clinic and one of her many roles is to counsel patients with food allergies and a need for healthy, anti-inflammatory diets. Jaclyn is a Food Practitioner and Vice President of Healthy Farm, Plate, You, LLC.

Endnotes

[1] Public Health, "Public Health".
[2] Cancer Prevention Coalition, "U.S. National Cancer Institute Manipulates Cancer Statistics."
[3] Centers for Disease Control and Prevention, "Women and Heart Disease Fact."
[4] Diabetes Prevention and Control Coalition, "Diabetes Facts and Figures."
[5] Office on Women's Health, U.S. health and Human Services, "Menstruation and the Menstrual Cycle Fact Sheet."
[6] CCN Health, "Boys--like girls--hitting puberty earlier."
[7] Mercola, "Mental Disorders Skyrocket: Try This To Avoid Becoming The Next Victim."
[8] Euromonitor International, "Health and Wellness the Trillion Dollar Industry in 2017: Key Research Highlights."
[9] Centers for Disease Control and Prevention, "Overweight and Obesity Data and Statistics."
[10] Centers for Disease Control and Prevention, "Overweight and Obesity Data and Statistics."
[11] Eat Wild, "Getting Wild Nutrition from Modern Food."
[12] American Cancer Society, "Recombinant Bovine Growth Hormone."
[13] Keep Antibiotics Working, "The Basics: Antibiotic Resistance."
[14] Pesticide Action Network. "Pan Pesticides Database – Pesticide Products."
[15] U.S. Department of Agriculture, "Organic Labeling and Marketing Information Fact Sheet."
[16] United States Environmental Protection Agency. "Pesticide news story: EPA releases report containing latest estimates of pesticide use in the United States."
[17] United States Environmental Protection Agency. "Pesticide news story: EPA releases report containing latest estimates of pesticide use in the United States."
[18] Pesticide Action Network. "Pan Pesticides Database – Pesticide Products."
[19] Pesticide Action Network. "Pan Pesticides Database – Pesticide Products."
[20] Pesticide Action Network. "Industrial Agriculture."
[21] Organic Consumer Association. "Irradiation Facts."
[22] Non-GMO Project. "What is GMO."
[23] Environmental Working Group. "Food News."
[24] Price, *2013 Shopping Guide,* 45-49.
[25] PETA, "Animals used for food."
[26] Weber, *FOOD, INC,* 22-23.
[27] PETA, "Animals used for food."
[28] Food & Water Watch, "Fact Sheet What Research Shows."
[29] Eat Wild, "Health Benefits."
[30] Salatin, *Folks, This Aint Normal,* 275-76.
[31] Ramsden, "Grass Fed Beef."
[32] The Cornucopia Institute, "Natural Meat Labels Confuse Shoppers."
[33] Price, *2013 Shopping Guide,* 36-42.
[34] Safran, *Eating Animals, 133.*
[35] PETA, "Animals Used for Food."
[36] Safran, *Eating Animals, 48.*
[37] Safran, *Eating Animals, 48.*

[38] BBC News, "Bald chicken 'needs no plucking'."
[39] Environmental Science and Technology, "Feather Meal: A Previously Unrecognized Route for Reentry into the Food Supply of Multiple Pharmaceuticals and Personal Care Products (PPCPs)."
[40] Environmental Science and Technology, "Feather Meal: A Previously Unrecognized Route for Reentry into the Food Supply of Multiple Pharmaceuticals and Personal Care Products (PPCPs)."
[41] Food & Water Watch, "Labels that tell you a little."
[42] Safran, *Eating Animals*, 48.
[43] Food Safety News, "Russia bans U.S. poultry over chlorine."
[44] L.A. Times, "The hidden salt in chicken."
[45] Keep Antibiotics Working, "Basics."
[46] Keep Antibiotics Working, "Basics."
[47] Keep Antibiotics Working, "Basics."
[48] Price, *2013 Shopping* Guide, 30-35.
[49] Safran, *Eating Animals*, 35.
[50] Food & Water Watch, "Fishy Farms: The Government's Push for Factory Farms in our Oceans.
[51] Center for Food Safety, "GE Fish."
[52] Environmental Protection Agency, "Human Health Criteria - Methylmercury Fish Tissue Criterion."
[53] McCabe, *Sunfood Living*, 116.
[54] McCabe, *Sunfood Living*, 116.
[55] McCabe, *Sunfood Living*, 106.
[56] Seafood Watch, "Seafood Watch Pocket Guide."
[57] Seafood Watch, "Seafood Watch Pocket Guide."
[58] George Mateljan Foundation, "Soybeans."
[59] George Mateljan Foundation, "Soybeans."
[60] George Mateljan Foundation, "Soybeans."
[61] George Mateljan Foundation, "Soybeans."
[62] CCOF, "What Does Organic Mean?"
[63] Non-GMO Project, "Non-GMO food soybean seed breeding program."
[64] George Mateljan Foundation, "Soybeans."
[65] George Mateljan Foundation, "Soybeans."
[66] Dr. Weil, "Dr. Weil's Anti-inflammatory Food Pyramid."
[67] Cornucopia Institute, "Soy Scorecard."
[68] U.S. Department of Agriculture, "Census of Agriculture."
[69] Organic Consumers Association, "GMO Food, Antibiotic Laced Meat and High Fructose Corn Syrup Have Made the U.S. the Fattest Nation in History!"
[70] Farm Sanctuary, "Dairy Production on Factory Farms."
[71] Farm Sanctuary, "Dairy Production on Factory Farms."
[72] Linda Joyce Forristal, CTA, MTA, "Ultra-Pasteurized Milk."
[73] Cornucopia Institute, "Dairy Scorecard."
[lxxiv] Price, *2013 Shopping Guide*, 97.
[75] Safran, *Eating Animals*, 78-79.
[76] Safran, *Eating Animals*, 61.
[77] Food Safety News, "European Union bans battery cages for egg laying hens."
[78] Farm Sanctuary, "Chickens used for eggs."

[79] Safran, *Eating Animals*, 60.
[80] Mother Earth News, "Is Agribusiness Making Food Less Nutritious?"
[81] Safran, *Eating Animals*, 61.
[82] Mother Earth News, "Free-range versus pastured chicken and eggs."
[83] Safran, *Eating Animals*, 61.
[84] Huffington Post, "The Cruelest of All Factory Farm Products: Eggs from Caged Hens."
[85] Huffington, Post, "The Cruelest of All Factory Farm Products: Eggs from Caged Hens."
[86] Huffington, Post, "The Cruelest of All Factory Farm Products: Eggs from Caged Hens."
[87] Cornucopia Institute, "Egg Scorecard."
[88] Pollan, *Food Rules: Eater's Manual*, 15.
[89] Pollan, *Food Rules: Eater's Manual*, 17.
[90] Mayo Clinic, "High-fructose corn syrup."
[91] WebMD, "Trans-fats."
[92] American Academy of Environmental Medicine, "GMO."
[93] Cornucopia Institute, "DHA Online Guide."
[94] Price, *2013 Shopping Guide*, 62-63.
[95] Price, *2013 Shopping Guide*, 59-61.
[96] Non-GMO Project, "Non-GMO Guide."
[97] Cornucopia Institute, "Cereal Scorecard."
[98] Price, *2013 Shopping Guide*, 72-75.
[99] Price, *2013 Shopping Guide*, 72-75.
[100] Price, *2013 Shopping Guide*, 88-90.
[101] Price, *2013 Shopping Guide*, 88-90.
[102] Price, *2013 Shopping Guide*, 88-90.
[103] Cornucopia Institute, "Hexane Guides Bars."
[104] Price, *2013 Shopping Guide*, 88-90.
[105] Price, *2013 Shopping Guide*, 19-25.
[106] Price, *2013 Shopping Guide*, 94-95.
[107] Price, *2013 Shopping Guide*, 93.
[108] Harvard School of Public Health, "Sugary Drinks and Obesity Fact Sheet."
[109] Harvard School of Public Health, "How Sweet Is It."
[110] American Heart Association, "Sugars and Carbohydrates."
[111] Diabetes Health, "The Dangers of High Fructose Corn Syrup."
[112] Sustainable Table Food Program, "Additives."
[113] Washington Post, "High-Fructose Corn Syrup: Not So Sweet for the Planet."
[114] Price, *2013 Shopping Guide*, 98-99.
[115] Price, *2013 Shopping Guide*, 99-102.

Made in the USA
San Bernardino, CA
19 February 2014